Mentalizing and Group Analysis

Mentalizing and Group Analysis presents a synthesis of group analysis and Mentalization-Based Group Therapy (MBT-G).

Sigmund Karterud brings together writing from the course of a career in group analysis and mentalization, beginning with a new introduction outlining the compelling theoretical case for hybrid versions of group analysis and MBT-G. The book covers key themes and ideas, including the group self, authority and leadership and personality, and presents an example of a high-quality mentalization-based group therapy session. Karterud's work provides a route forward for the evolution of theory and practice of group analysis.

Mentalizing and Group Analysis will be of great interest to group psychotherapists and group analysts in practice and in training.

Sigmund Karterud, MD, PhD is professor of psychiatry, formerly at the University of Oslo, founder of The Norwegian Institute for Mentalization, a former training group analyst at Institute of Group Analysis, Oslo and member of Group Analytic Society International (GASi). He has published widely on themes related to group analysis, maintains a private practice in Oslo and supervises and lectures internationally.

The New International Library of Group Analysis (NILGA)

Series Editor: Earl Hopper

Drawing on the seminal ideas of British, European and American group analysts, psychoanalysts, social psychologists and social scientists, the books in this series focus on the study of small and large groups, organisations and other social systems, and on the study of the transpersonal and transgenerational sociality of human nature. NILGA books will be required reading for the members of professional organisations in the field of group analysis, psychoanalysis, and related social sciences. They will be indispensable for the "formation" of students of psychotherapy, whether they are mainly interested in clinical work with patients or in consultancy to teams and organisational clients within the private and public sectors.

Recent titles in the series include:

Group Analysis
A Modern Synthesis
Sigmund Karterud

Tolerance – A Concept in Crisis
Psychoanalytic, Group Analytic, and Socio-Cultural Perspectives
Edited by Avi Berman and Gila Ofer

Advances in Group Psychotherapy
Living in the Passionate Bad Fit
Stewart L. Aledort, Edited by Lee Kassan

The Power of Group Attachment
John Bowlby Revisited from a Group-Analytic Perspective
Arturo Ezquerro and María Cañete

Mentalizing and Group Analysis
Sigmund Karterud

"This book offers a truly thrilling experience for those interested in wanting to know how Group Analysis can benefit from mentalization theories. It dives deep into different theoretical contexts, showing how they all have contributed to the development of mentalization concepts that can enrich and expand group analysis in theory and practice. A book that finally can explain, why mentalization concepts are absolutely necessary, if Group Analysis wants to grow and catch up with modern times."– **Prof. Dr. Elisabeth Rohr, Philipps-Universität Marburg/Germany, training group analyst and international consultant**

"This book, by one of the foremost pioneers of mentalizing, offers a magisterial account of the centrality of group processes in mentalization-based therapy. It builds a brilliant bridge between group analysis and mentalizing, showing with great clarity how the recovery of mentalizing depends not only on the individual but on the shared experience of the group, and how theories of social communication are integral to our understanding of mentalizing itself. Extending the discourse from Freud and Foulkes to modern group analysis to social ontology, the author provides profound insights into the mentalizing processes of groups while never losing sight of clinical relevance. This is a remarkable achievement: a work of deep scholarship that will also transform everyday therapeutic practice." – **Professor Peter Fonagy CBE FMedSci FBA FAcSS; Head of the Division of Psychology and Language Sciences National Clinical Advisor on Children's Mental Health, NHS England, University College, London**

"This book by Sigmund Karterud makes an outstanding contribution to both the theory and practice of group psychotherapy. By bringing together the concepts of mentalization and group analysis, Karterud offers a fresh, integrative framework that deepens our understanding of how groups foster self-reflection, empathy, and interpersonal learning. With clinical wisdom and theoretical clarity, he demonstrates how mentalizing processes unfold within group dynamics and how therapists can cultivate them to enhance therapeutic effectiveness. This volume is essential reading not only for group analysts but also for all psychotherapists who wish to better grasp the relational mind and the transformative potential of groups." – **Haim Weinberg, PhD, licensed psychologist and group analyst. Sacramento Center for Psychotherapy.**

"While the volume as a whole is rooted in psychotherapy and mentalization-based treatment, its opening chapter makes a particularly significant contribution by situating group analysis within a broader social and organizational frame. In fact, *Mentalizing and Group Analysis* is a landmark contribution that refreshes and repositions group analysis within the wider landscape of contemporary social and organizational life. By weaving together mentalization theory, linguistic philosophy, and group analytic tradition, Sigmund Karterud demonstrates how groups function not merely as therapeutic instruments but as living spaces where meaning, identity, and cooperation are continually negotiated. This perspective expands the value of group analysis beyond psychotherapy: it shows its relevance for understanding organizational cultures, intergroup tensions, and collective responses to uncertainty. At a time when institutions face profound challenges, this chapter provides an intellectual framework and a practical compass for fostering reflective, resilient, and genuinely communicative groups in professional and societal contexts." – **Roberta Mineo, Ph.D. Tenured academic, Department of Humanities, University of Modena and Reggio Emilia, Italy**

"Fascinating. In recent years, MBT has further distinguished itself by drawing upon diverse developmental sciences and cognitive neuroscience. Sigmund Karterud has developed his own distinctive work, focusing on MBT-G and seeking to discuss it integrally with Group Analysis. It is highly unique. The author's erudition enabled the discussion to encompass a broad range of fields, including philosophy and linguistics, rendering it incredibly rich. The co-authored work with Walter Stone, which discusses group through self-psychology theory, is impressive. There is the meticulous empirical research on MBT group, which contributes to clarifying MBT-G's significance. Then he sheds new light on Group Analysis through MBT. Finally, the convergence of both strands successfully opens new horizons for group therapy. My respect to the authors." – **Kaoru Nishimura, Professor, International Christian University, Japan; Vice president, Japanese Association for Group Psychotherapy; Former Board Member, International Association for Group Psychotherapy and Group Processes (IAGP)**

"Bringing discussions on linguistics turn in philosophy, the dialectics between matter and mind, nature and culture, social ontology, as well as in classic and contemporary authors in psychoanalysis and group analysis, Sigmund Karterud brings an interesting dialogue between Mentalization-Based Group Therapy (MBT-G) and the theory and practice of group analysis. Through theoretical inputs and clinical vignettes, the book illustrates how MBT-G is a contemporary, relevant and effective contribution to group treatment of "patients difficult to reach", especially patients with borderline and personality disorders. In this direction, the MBT-G theory and technique are a fundamental tool to face contemporary patients' mental health struggles." – **Carla Penna, PhD, psychoanalyst and group analyst in Brazil. She is a member of the Group Analytic Society International and IAGP. She is a former president of the Brazilian Association of Group Psychotherapy and a former Visiting Professor of Medical Psychology at the University State of Rio de Janeiro**

Mentalizing and Group Analysis by Sigmund Karterud is a landmark contribution to contemporary psychoanalytic and group analytic literature. This volume builds on the author's extensive previous work in mentalization-based treatment (MBT-G) and classical group analysis, offering a rigorous and innovative integration of the two. What distinguishes this text is its depth of theoretical insight combined with an empirically grounded clinical vision that enhances the field's capacity to treat increasingly complex psychopathologies. Karterud's core thesis, that the capacity for mentalizing is not only an intrapsychic function but a deeply relational and group-dependent process, is as timely as it is necessary. The author presents a compelling argument that group analytic processes are inherently mentalizing when facilitated with clinical skill and theoretical awareness. The text re-centres the therapeutic group as a space for symbolization, co-construction of meaning, and affective transformation. This reconceptualization echoes the radical insights of S. H. Foulkes, extending them into a relational and linguistically attuned framework aligned with contemporary philosophy and social ontology. In an age of increasing fragmentation within the field, Karterud's synthesis bridges individual and collective dimensions of psychic life, offering a robust model that speaks to the "group mind" without falling into reification. His critique of outdated constructs, such as the traditional "group mind," and his redefinition of the "group matrix" through the lens of intersubjectivity, language, and evolution, marks a crucial advancement in group analytic thought. Equally significant is the empirical grounding of the book. Drawing on published research and video discourse studies from actual group sessions, including work with borderline patients, Karterud demonstrates how theory can be meaningfully applied to clinical practice. His writing remains accessible without sacrificing intellectual rigor, making it an essential text for group analysts, relational psychoanalysts, and clinicians working with severe personality disorders. This book is not merely a commentary on existing paradigms; it is a bold proposal for the future of psychoanalysis and psychotherapy. It invites the reader into a dialogical and evolving tradition of thought, one that honors its historical foundations while courageously stepping into new terrain. *Mentalizing and Group Analysis* deserves to become a foundational text in the training of group therapists, supervisors, and relational psychoanalytic scholars worldwide." – **Stavros Charalambides, CGP, MSc. Director, Institute for Relational & Group Psychotherapy, Athens**

Mentalizing and Group Analysis

Sigmund Karterud

Routledge
Taylor & Francis Group
LONDON AND NEW YORK

Designed cover image: © Getty Images

First published 2026
by Routledge
4 Park Square, Milton Park, Abingdon, Oxon OX14 4RN

and by Routledge
605 Third Avenue, New York, NY 10158

Routledge is an imprint of the Taylor & Francis Group, an informa business

British Library Cataloguing-in-Publication Data
A catalogue record for this book is available from the British Library

ISBN: 9781041038788 (hbk)
ISBN: 9781041038771 (pbk)
ISBN: 9781003625810 (ebk)

DOI: 10.4324/9781003625810

Typeset in Times New Roman
by Newgen Publishing UK

For Birgit and Marianne

Contents

Foreword

This volume relates to my previous books *Mentalization-Based Group Therapy (MBT-G): A Theoretical, Clinical and Research Manual (2015)* and *Group Analysis. A Modern Synthesis (2023).* The first one is very much "applied" group analysis, while the second is about group analysis in a more classical sense. In this book, my point of departure is the very concept of mentalizing. Although there is something labelled mentalization-based treatment (MBT), the concept of mentalizing need not imply any specific therapeutic method. Mentalizing refers to how subjective experiences can be symbolised and thought about within a human group/society, and the prerequisites and qualities of such thinking. In particular it is about meaning-formation of intersubjective experiences. A central tenet is that mentalizing presupposes a group which is capable of thinking about collective affairs (intentionality). I suggest that these ideas shed new light on the communicational processes in therapeutic groups, which was the primary concern of S. H. Foulkes (1948, 1964) in his theory and practice of group analysis. Thus, I discuss the significance of mentalizing theory for the theory and conduct of group analysis. This is the more practical aim which also has clear implications for the treatment of e.g., personality disorders (Karterud, 2015). However, I suggest that the theory of mentalizing, when seen as part of the linguistic turn in philosophy, also has radical implications for the understanding of questions like what the nature of groups is, if the concept of a group mind is meaningful, and the need for a redefinition of the concept group matrix. That composes the first essay.

The following chapters are based upon articles published in the journal *Group Analysis* and *International Journal of Group Psychotherapy* during the years 2003–2024. While the introduction is mainly conceptual and philosophical, the subsequent articles try to demonstrate the clinical relevance through empirical studies. The articles are the following:

Karterud, S. & Stone, W. N. (2003). The group self: A neglected aspect of group psychotherapy. *Group Analysis*, 36(1): 7–22.

Stone, W. N. & Karterud, S. (2006). Dreams as portraits of self and group interaction. *International Journal of Group Psychotherapy*, 56(1): 47–62, 2006.

Karterud, S. (2012). Constructing and Mentalizing the Matrix. *Group Analysis*, 44(4): 357–373.

Inderhaug, T. & Karterud, S. (2015). A qualitative study of a mentalization-based group for borderline patients. *Group Analysis*, 48(2): 150–163.

Karterud, S. (2015). On structure and leadership in MBT-G and group analysis. *Group Analysis*, 48(2): 137–149.

Kalleklev, J. & Karterud, S. (2018). A comparative study of a mentalization-based versus a psychodynamic group therapy session. *Group Analysis*, 51(1): 44–60.

Karterud, S. (2018). A high-quality mentalization-based group therapy session. *Group Analysis*, 51(1): 18–43.

Karterud, S., Folmo, E. & Kongerslev, M. T. (2019). Personality and the group matrix. *Group Analysis*, 52(4), DOI: 10.1177/0533316418824210.

Karterud, S., Gunnarsen, G., Kongerslev, M. T., Staun, L. & Schultz-Venrath, U. (2024). On the relationship between group analysis and mentalization-based group therapy. *Group Analysis*, 58(1), DOI: 10.1177/05333164231218694

I thank the journals for letting me reproduce these texts, as well as my co-authoring colleagues Walter Stone, Tryggve Inderhaug, Jens Kalleklev, Espen Folmo, Mickey Kongerslev, Gunnar Gunnarsen, Lenka Staun and Ulrich Schultz-Venrath. Together we have done a lot of interesting work on theory and detailed discourse studies of video-recorded group sessions. In Norway, I belong to the Norwegian Institute for Group Analysis and Group Psychotherapy (IGA) and to the Norwegian Institute for Mentalization. There I run theory seminars and training courses. And, together with my colleagues at the Psychotherapy Laboratory at Oslo University Hospital, I am engaged in refining our scales for group psychotherapy ratings. A lot of colleagues have thus contributed to the development of the ideas brought forward in this book. Besides my co-authors I would like to mention Malcolm Pines, Paul Ornstein, Anthony Bateman, Peter Fonagy, Thor Kristian Island, Steinar Lorentzen, Theresa Wilberg, Øyvind Urnes, Siri Johns, Synnøve Ness-Bjerke, Hanne Sofie Dahl, Audun Ulland, Tone Normann-Eide, Andreas Ekberg, Kjetil Bremer, Finn Skårderud, Bente Sommerfeldt and Henning Jordet. A special thanks goes to Earl Hopper who supported this work and was helpful with editing and composing the text.

Oslo, September 2025
Sigmund Karterud

Chapter 1

Mentalizing and group analysis

Sigmund Karterud

Abstract

In this introductory essay the author claims that the theory of mentalizing is a necessary component of the theory and practice of group analysis, and vice versa that group analysis might enrich the theory of mentalizing by extending it beyond a two-person psychology. The essay situates the theory of mentalizing as part of a psychoanalytic discourse on the origin and function of thoughts, with references to Sigmund Freud and Wilfred Bion, and part of a linguistic turn in philosophy that claims that language constitutes the social world, with references to Charles Taylor and John Searle. These perspectives expand group analytic theory, as outlined by S. H. Foulkes, and strengthen his theory of communication and the role of the group analyst as a co-creator of a certain type of therapeutic group discourse which enables a transformation of symptoms, such as unmentalized emotions, located at the level of the individuals. Furthermore, the author argues that the concept of group mind should be abandoned and that the concept of group matrix should be redefined with references to modern theories of evolution, emotions, attachment, mentalizing, as well as social ontology (Searle). In summary, it is contended that such a clarification and redefinition of the foundation of group analysis might favour a more flexible approach to the benefit of clients with more serious personality problems as found in public mental health services.

Psychoanalysis and group analysis are theoretical systems and practices in perpetual development. They will never reach any permanent conclusion. They are not like mathematical formulas, like 2 + 2 = 4, which were true 2000 years ago and still are true today. They are evolving and changing systems; since people change, and cultures change, there would therefore also be a change in the way we interpret human affairs. They are situated in history in a radically different way than mathematical formulas. They evolve out of history, take on their distinct persona through the grounding conceptualizations, impact history and eventually become transcended by history.

The purpose of this introductory essay is to discuss how the modern concept of mentalizing has changed, or will change, the theory and practice of group analysis.

DOI: 10.4324/9781003625810-1

Hopefully, there is a dialectics here, that this discussion also will deepen our understanding of what mentalizing is all about.

Our history starts around the end of World War II. Europe is liberated from tyranny. There is a feeling of euphoria, of victory, of hope and optimism for the future, and above all a feeling of freedom. Tyranny in the outer world has been fought down. The new terrain to be conquered is the souls of the battered that carry wounds from past experiences and submission to internal oppressors. Therapeutic communities in the United Kingdom are important sites. *Free and open communication* is the foremost slogan, in small and large groups and through the institutions themselves. The English pioneer Tom Main (1946) proclaimed, "The hospital as doctor" through a "culture of enquiry" (Karterud, 1996). By such means, the individual would heal his/her wounds and restore personal dignity.

Early in the history of group analysis, S. H. Foulkes (1948, 1957) highlighted this free and open communication. The main task of the group analyst was not so much that of presenting interpretations as in classical psychoanalysis, but to analyse the ongoing group process to liberate the communicational flow which could be stuck in the individual, between people or by systemic forces in the group as a whole. Foulkes suggested music metaphors for therapeutic group dynamics. He likened the role of the therapist to that of a *conductor* of an orchestra and coined the concept of *resonance* in groups. He maintained that optimally, the painful and warded off parts in the individual would create some kind of response in other group members. By their resonance, the painful experiences of the individual might find a new route for becoming symbolized and expressed verbally. However, this process required skilful handling of the group processes by the group analyst, above all a *translation.* The group analyst should translate distorted communication to commonsense language whereby the resources of the surrounding culture could be mobilized. The relationship individual-group-society was conceptualized through the notion of a *group matrix* which was the mostly unconscious communicational web that connected individual persons in groups and societies. Societies were bound together by *foundational matrices* which consisted of a common language, history and culture, while smaller groups for specific purposes were united by *dynamic matrices* reflecting their tasks, resources and constraints. *Personal matrices* reflected the personality makeup of the individual. These matrices harboured interacting forces. According to Foulkes (1964), forces in the foundation and dynamic matrix would *penetrate the individual* to the innermost core. The individual could be *likened to a nod* in these dynamic systems. Notwithstanding the complexity of these systems, Foulkes maintained that they were civilized or had a potential for civilization. There was always a possibility for liberating prosocial forces in the matrix that might help overcome *emotional blockages in the personal matrix* of the individual. Foulkes held an *optimistic view* of healing potentials in therapeutic groups.

The conceptualizations that I have referred to above were far ahead of psychoanalysis at that time. They were radical. At the same time, Foulkes considered himself a psychoanalyst of a "strictly Freudian persuasion". This contradiction was later to be referred to as the "radical Foulkes" versus the "conservative Foulkes" (Dalal, 1998). The idea that there are forces in the individual that is kept out of consciousness because their liberation would threaten the balance and integrity and thus frighten the person, was not radical. That is plain drive theory and ego psychology. It was maintained that it is the nature of drives that they seek for discharge, and it is the nature of the ego that it searches for compromises between drive expressions and social order through the regulating function of the superego. However, this rather solipsistic psychic apparatus view of the nature of man came with limited explanatory power and restricted freedom for the practicing analyst. Ego psychology was bound to be transcended, both for theoretical and therapeutic reasons. The Zeitgeist in the 20th century moved relentlessly in the direction of relational theories and practices (Kohut, 1977; Mitchell, 1998).

Foulkes may be considered a pioneer in relational psychoanalysis. And a very radical one too, since what he emphasized were relations between ordinary people in a certain social setting, not the relation between an empathic psychological expert and a suffering individual. A considerable problem, however was the fact that although his theory was "correct" in some sense, it was not spelled out in detail. To a certain extent, *it lacked a more profound grounding.* This incompleteness of group analytic theory has been emphasized by many authors (e.g., Malcolm Pines, John Schlapobersky). Let me hasten to comment here, with reference to the remarks at the beginning of this chapter, that group analytic theory will never be "completed". However, it may become more coherent, richer, more in tune and in dialogue with neighbouring disciplines (like philosophy, evolution and personality theory) and thus become more robust and useful for psychopathologies of modern times.

It is a thesis in this book that the concept of mentalizing might consolidate group analytic theory and pave way for a more flexible practice. This is so because it concerns the essence of group analysis, which is symbolization and verbalization through resonance in several minds during psychotherapeutic group processes that promote self and personality development. By that it also concerns the dialectics of matter and mind, nature and culture. For example, how can nature be converted to culture? It concerns the very process of civilization. As such, it demands an evolutionary perspective. How and when did civilization arise? What were the decisive evolutionary processes? I have discussed these questions in my book *Group Analysis. A Modern Synthesis* (Karterud, 2023). Here I go more in depth. In particular when it comes to the notion of *man as a language animal* (Taylor, 2016) and its implications.

The practical implications concern the challenges that come with personality disorders in our time. Almost by definition, persons with different degrees and types of personality disorders present with complex mentalizing problems (Fonagy et al., 2002). For many of them, these problems affect their identity as a disturbing confusion about the sense of self. Thus, in a very practical sense, we become faced with the problem of self and subjectivity for the conduct of group analysis. It also concerns the group as constituted by collective intentionality. We cannot avoid the question of the group self. In the second and more empirical part of this book, based upon published papers, I will discuss therapeutic challenges due to self, personality and mentalizing disturbances in concert with the group self, group culture and group discourse.

Thinking, language and mentalizing

The concept of mentalizing has a short and a longer history. The landmark volume in modern times was Peter Fonagy and coworkers' book (2002) *Affect regulation, mentalization and the development of the self.* The title is noteworthy. It points to the significance of affects and mentalization for the development of the self. We are not talking about the ego any longer, but the self. We are not talking about a part of a psychic apparatus, but the self as the existential core of the person. The authors follow in the footsteps of the psychoanalytic master of the self, Heinz Kohut (1971, 1977), and the pioneer of empirical studies of self-development, Daniel Stern (1985). However, they go "deeper", into the very building blocks of the self. How does nature become culture?

They lean on a longer psychoanalytic history. Sigmund Freud was from the very beginning impressed by *the forces of the body-mind.* Hysterical symptoms witnessed about powerful forces. What was their nature? Freud's theory of drives said that drives sought outlet, or *discharge* as was his terminology. However, according to Freud (1895/1966), the drives, as somatic excitations, risk wild and disorganized discharge, to the detriment of the individual. He postulated a bio-psycho-economic origin of thought, whereby thought exerted a "Bindung" (linking and binding) effect upon somatic excitation. This Bindung linked somatic excitation (drive) and thought and enabled a secondary inhibitory process which made representation (and thinking) of the absent object (for the drives) possible. These ideas were developed in detail in his book *Project for a Scientific Psychology* (written in 1895 but not published until 1950) which founded essential parts of his metapsychology. What we consider here is his reflections about thinking. His primary interest was in the *function* of thought and thinking and he stated that they were in the service of taming the wild drives. He speculated how thoughts could do this job on the level of the neuron. He did not discuss where thoughts came from, e.g., their relations to words, concepts and meaning. He took that for granted. Furthermore, he postulated *unconscious thoughts* that operated on the neuronal level. There was the location, so to speak, where nature was converted to culture. When neuronal drive excitation was bound by thought, thinking could occur with these thoughts at the level of the ego and thereby becoming modified by the reality principles of logic and reason.

The most obvious problem with this reasoning is the confusion of discourse. Freud started his career in the field of neurology and performed research upon neuronal activity. That was a new and promising field in the late 1800 century. Neurons could be identified as (miniscule) objects in the world and thus be investigated by methods of natural sciences. However, "thoughts" do not belong to that kind of discourse. Thoughts cannot be measured in the same way. It is meaningless to state that a thought can "bind" neuronal excitation, unless one speaks in metaphorical ways. However, Freud meant it not as metaphors, but literally. That creates confusion. Today we would say that of course, "thoughts" do not bind neuronal excitation, but certain synaptic activity might "bind" neuronal excitation. As an example benzodiazepine medication will activate the gamma-butyric-acid system which will reduce neuronal glutamate excitation and thereby calm down the *emotional system of fear* (in Freuds words "curbing wild and disorganized discharge"). Today we also know that the same effect can be achieved, e.g., curbing a panic attack, by comfort, since comfort also works through hormonal and transmitter systems that involve the gamma-butyric-acid system.

Since the *Project* was unpublished until 1950, the content of this volume was not much debated among psychoanalysts before the thorough volume of Pribram & Gill (1976), *Freud's "Project" Re-assessed.* However, Wilfred Bion addressed the same theme in a series of books and papers from the late 1950s and 1960s (Bion, 1962, 1963, 1965, 1967a, 1967b). Bion was no neurologist and did not follow Freud on the neuronal path but expanded the ideas of *unconscious thoughts.* Bion developed a kind of discourse that was quite original, where he tried to find another path than the natural-scientific on the one hand (neuronal excitation) or the humanistic-hermeneutic on the other hand (thoughts as carriers of meaning). He invented an idiosyncratic discourse filled with metaphors like beta-elements, alfa-elements, alfa-function, evacuation, container, contained, -K (against knowledge) and L (love), etc. He aimed at developing a system to understand the thinking mind that would be like mathematical systems or the periodic system of natural elements. He spoke and wrote in a manner that obscured the question of metaphors versus objective reality. Beta-elements, where they palpable elements, or were they just metaphorical concepts? Bion would say they were both (!) They were metaphors that might be filled with objective meaning along the course of scientific development.

According to Bion, beta-elements were personal sense impressions or so-called pre-conceptions, which were not yet available for thinking. Beta-elements had to undergo a process of so-called alfa-function to be converted into alfa-elements, which had the qualities of thoughts which made them suitable to be processed by the mental operation of thinking, and whereby the reality principle could exert its influence. Beta-elements could not be thought about, they could just be evacuated from the mind. This was the essence of the paranoid-schizoid position, according to Bion. This highly mechanical way of reasoning lead to the next question, which was about the space into which these beta-elements could be evacuated. The optimal fate, according to Bion, was an evacuation into a container that could perform an alfa-function by proxy so to speak (so-called reverie) which made it possible to re-introject the evacuated beta-elements into a transformed state and turned into alfa-elements which now could be thought about by the protagonist. In worst case, the beta-elements could get even more bizarre and alien and render the protagonist in a state of "nameless dread". The optimal fate would depend upon a "good breast-container-mother", the worst case involved a "bad and persecutory breast-container-mother".

Thinking, according to Bion, is a function that develops in the individual to handle alfa-elements (thoughts), and which protects the individual from madness (being overwhelmed by unmetabolized beta-elements). It needs to be added that Bion's theoretical system included the existence of so-called pre-conceptions. This is a line of thought that can be traced back to Freud's "Totem and Taboo" (1913) where Freud (erroneously) postulated that personal experiences (e.g., with the Oedipus conflict) could alter the genetic code and be transferred to next generations (e.g., as taboo conceptions and taboo behaviour). In a similar way, Bion claimed that the baby had a pre-conception of a breast. When the baby had an encounter with the breast, either positive or negative, the pre-conception of the breast might be transformed into a concept of the breast which could be thought about. And in a similar way, that the encounter with the father would activate the inborn pre-conception of the Oedipal constellation.

It is necessary to devote some space to Bion's theories since they have influenced to a considerable degree our thinking about group dynamics (Bion, 1961). As I have tried to demonstrate, he followed clearly in Freud's footsteps. Both claimed that the main function of thoughts and thinking was to prevent man becoming a victim of madness due to the overwhelming discharge pressure from potentially destructive drives (beta-elements). Freud's discourse was mainly intrapsychic, while Bion was a pioneer for the next object-relational generation since he introduced the concept of a container (another person/mind = "object") as a necessary means for thought formation. Unfortunately, both were bound to a mechanical universe (which also influenced Foulkes in his way of thinking about the mind and matrix). Freud spoke in a very concrete way about thoughts exerting a kind of Bindung, similar to the function of benzodiazepines upon glutamate neuronal activation, and Bion spoke about "elements" being converted to other kind of elements through some mysterious function of something labelled "reverie" performed by a "container". We should consider these concepts borrowed from mechanical systems as metaphors. However, the problem is that the authors themselves meant it in an almost (?) literal manner and that later generations of scholars and practitioners were confused as to what is metaphorical and what is literal. Freud himself had considerable doubt about the fruitfulness of his "Project" and decided not to publish his manuscript. He realized that he was writing about a topic that was dependent upon neurophysiological progress and he changed his orientation towards a "pure psychology". However, the way of reasoning which he developed in the "Project" was to be continued in his later metapsychology. Bion never left his speculative theory of thinking although it never got any hold outside some circles of psychoanalysis. Although Bion had an idea of making psychoanalysis more "scientific" by suggesting a classification system for thoughts and thought processes, he turned more and more into a "mystic" (Bion, 1975).

Among the many problems with Freud's and Bion's ideas of thoughts and thinking, I would like to emphasize not only the lack of evolutionary perspectives but also their faulty evolutionary reasoning. Both adhered to Lamarcanian ideation, i.e., that personal experiences might be inherited, which is opposed to Darwin's concept of natural selection due to survival fitness. In addition, they lacked any theory of language and language development, and particularly any theory of the evolution of language. Instead they proposed the highly speculative idea, not founded in any scientific study of language development, that thoughts and thinking developed as means to avoid madness and that the psychoanalytic study of madness (ref Bion's writings on psychoses, Bion, 1967) would be the road to understanding the nature of thinking. This implies that the true nature of certain phenomena can only be obtained by a study of pathological versions of the same phenomena, e.g., the true nature of how the heart functions can be obtained by studying diseased hearts instead of studying normal and well-functioning hearts. I would also add the problem of *discussing these issues at the level of words.* Isolated words, words in themselves, are meaningless. Words get their meanings by reference to the language of which they are a part. Words can calm us down, e.g., suppress neuronal excitation, not because the words act on the synapses in the same way as a diazepam pill does, but because they might *convey meanings* which are essential to us.

Michael Tomasello (2014, 2019) is a relevant modern researcher who has studied and constructed an evolutionary based theory of language and thinking. Tomasello starts with the phenomenon of communication. Homo sapiens is not the only species that communicates. However, Homo sapiens do that in a far more sophisticated manner than other species. The most important outcome of good communication is *better cooperation* between individuals, which represents *survival values*. Better communication might also have the benefit of protecting people against madness, but that is not the *reason* why it evolved. It evolved because it, e.g., made people cooperate better when hunting together and being able to share the hunting prey in a manner that benefitted all the involved families as well as the village to which they belonged. Sophisticated hunting demanded sophisticated communication (e.g., the building of hunting pits) which required an understanding of the intentions of the hunting comrades. What's going on in their minds? Are they committed to this hunting project? Do they understand what I'm trying to communicate? Do they *understand my intentions*? The more sophisticated words and concepts and language, the better people will cooperate and the less misunderstandings. The better clarification and mutual problem solving. To achieve that, their words, concepts and language should not be private communicational signals but grounded in a system that they, as a group, had agreed upon. By that, they could also move from personal, individual intentions, to *collective intentions*. They could perform actions on behalf of the group since they had the ability to share and discuss common interests through a language which was meaningful to everybody. In fact, meaning is constituted through this language, and words get their meaning with reference to other words and concepts in the language system.

Among all the wonderful things we can do with a language, we may develop the ability to understand, not only the intentions of others and how the external world functions, but also ourselves. As such, language is a presupposition for coming to know oneself, i.e., for self-consciousness. Language is predominately a group phenomenon and in a certain respect it is correct to say that the group is prior to the individual. Without a conversing group, there would be no person in a modern sense which could think and reflect and situate him/herself in a given social context. There would be primitive individuals who could cooperate around the most basic life necessities, but there would not be self-consciousness in our meaning of the term. Those individuals would have self-awareness but quite limited self-consciousness.

The reader may have noticed how the present discourse has moved from thoughts and thinking to the concepts of self and consciousness. This brings us back to history, e.g., to the development of ideas in the wake of Bion in London during the 1970s and 1980s. While Bion never reached out of marginal psychoanalytic communities, his rival John Bowlby, who early on became an outsider in the British psychoanalytic community, raised to be a founder of a new paradigm with his theory of *attachment* (Bowlby, 1969, 1973, 1980). In our days, attachment is embraced by "everybody". The main difference between the two British psychoanalysts, living in the same city at the same time, was that Bion followed a course of metapsychology and tried to capture the essence of man through psychopathological concepts, while Bowlby followed an empirical path and tried to find the essence of man in concepts of normal functioning. According to Bowlby (1969), the normal path of the baby, and which baby and mother are both designed for, is to become attached to the caregiver. But sometimes this attachment process might go wrong. And this unfortunate development can be measured empirically by observational methods. That is how the *"Strange Situation Test"* of Mary Ainsworth (and John Bowlby) came to be developed (Ainsworth, Blehar, Waters, & Wall, 2015). The success of the Strange Situation Test prompted Mary Main to develop another test for classifying attachment patterns among adults, the *"Adult Attachment Interview"* (George, Main, & Kaplan, 1985). Children could be observed in a stressful situation where they were exposed to strangers (fear) and experienced separation anxiety when their mothers left the room. Their behaviour could thus be classified. Adults can cope with such a situation despite different attachment patterns. A different method was needed to determine the attachment pattern of adults. A special type of interview was the answer.

The Adult Attachment Interview (AAI) was designed as to "*challenge the unconscious*" by a series of questions about the childhood experiences of the protagonist. When rating the interview, the raters should judge the *quality of the protagonist's discourse*. Most notably, the criteria for this judgment were inspired by the theories of the British philosopher Paul Grice (1989). Grice was a pioneer of linguistic philosophy, emphasizing the pragmatics of ordinary language. He underlined communication as a basically cooperative endeavour and formulated a set of maxims for sound communication:

- A maxim of quantity: 1) Be as informative as necessary (for the purpose of the discourse); 2) Do not be more informative than necessary.
- A maxim of quality: Be truthful. 1) Do not say anything you believe to be untrue; 2) Do not say anything which you cannot verify.
- A maxim of relation and balance: Be relevant.
- A maxim of means: Be clear. 1) Avoid unclear formulations; 2) Avoid ambiguities; 3) Be concise (avoid redundant and conspicuous wordplay); 4) Be organized.

The thesis (which was confirmed by a series of studies) was that individuals with insecure attachment patterns contained painful memories which, when evoked, were difficult to speak about in a clearcut manner (Cassidy & Shaver, 1999). These memories had not been reorganized and processed along with later socio-cognitive personality development. They had not been transformed along with maturation, which we might express in ego-psychological terms like not being modified by the reality principle because these painful memories were partly unconscious. *Accordingly, when the protagonist was asked to speak about these memories, s/he might respond by words and sentences that signalled unintegrated emotions, contradictions, lack of reflections, lack of complexity, simplicity, lack of memories and words, a confusing syntax, etc.* When Peter Fonagy joined this research field, he and coworkers became particularly interested in the questions in the AAI that "demanded" a so-called "mentalizing response". E.g., questions like "what's your thoughts about why your parents did X?" Demand questions asked about *opinions about intentionality* and tested the quality of these responses according to Grice's maxims for sound communication. Were the responses informative, truthful, relevant and clear? This work led to the manual for testing, *Reflective Functioning,* which became the definition of mentalizing (Fonagy et al., 1998). The protagonist's responses to demand questions were rated on a scale from -1 to 9. A rating of 9 indicated excellent mentalizing ability (e.g., complex, rich, thoughtful answers containing many perspectives), while a negative rating of -1 indicated very poor mentalizing ability, bordering at psychotic functioning with e.g., bizarre utterances, denials, serious contradictions, hostility or delusionary thinking. The level of everyday good enough reflective functioning was set to a rating level of 5. Below that level, the individual would encounter increasing problems in communication with others and a series of misunderstandings of others as well as him/herself with negative consequences for interpersonal and intrapsychic functioning.

The history of ideas which I have described (all too briefly) developed from some confusing ideas (Freud) about thoughts being able to influence directly upon neuronal activity (excitation), to precursors of thoughts (Bion) being "modified by a container", to empirical studies of speech acts (Fonagy), relying on a pragmatic philosophy of language. The latter position acknowledges that language exists prior to the ontogenesis of the individual and that it has evolved as means of communication for the purpose of human cooperation which is fundamental to civilization. The latter is a far more positive view on civilization than what Freud (1930) expressed in his volume "Civilization and its discontents". It also implies that language becomes far more than a "means of communication".

We can trace this philosophical tradition back to Georg Hegel (1807/2019), being considerably developed by different philosophers like Paul Grice, Paul Ricoeur, Charles Taylor and John Searle. Their theories have profound implications for what we mean by words, concepts and phenomena like self, consciousness and social world. Most important is the thesis that *language constitutes the social world* (Taylor, 2016). There will of course exist a world without language which is inhabited by speechless animals, but there would be nobody to say the word "world", not to speak of the words of "love", "envy" and "gratitude". Non-human animals are conscious about the world, in that they experience the world and behave rational in this world according to their own logic and modes of communication. They do not ramble around at random. They beset a *core self* that organizes experience and is the source of actions. And many mammals of these animals live in families and groups. However, these animal groups are not *spiritual groups*, with reference to Hegel (1807/2019). They are not organized around *constitutive speech acts* that define the rules and regulations of the groups and their dynamics. *Such constitutive speech acts (Searle, 2010; Taylor, 2016; Tomasello, 2019) depend on the existence (through evolution) of linguistic conventions which are grounded in collective intentionality.* In an evolutionary sense, there develops a "we" which is grounded upon collective agreements on words, concepts and grammar, as well as behavioural rules and regulations that carry some kind of ethics and morality. *Furthermore, this we, this collective agreement, become bound to a history which can be narrated.* Hegel was quite sceptical of the profoundness of civilizations that rested upon oral traditions alone. He said that such civilizations lacked any history proper, which he claimed depended upon *written discourses*. A proper development of the Spirit (as discussed in the *Phenomenology of the Spirit*, Hegel 1807) could only take place through the discussions of written texts. Later we will come back to the implications of Searle's views for the very concept and existence of the social phenomenon "group" and thereby the concept of matrix.

In modern terms, the ongoing dynamics of the Zeitgeist is negotiated in media and educational agencies like universities which contain databases and libraries of written texts and recordings of speech and visual images. For the Spirit to develop, oral exchange must be objectified. That is also a central claim by Paul Ricoeur (1981) when he discussed the scientific grounds of the humanities. Phenomenology is not enough, said Ricoeur. Hermeneutics is the answer, according to Ricoeur, and it *transcends the artificial boundaries between the natural sciences and the humanities*. The historical roots of hermeneutics are the problems of interpretations of the Bible. The Bible is a "grounding" document for a whole civilization. It contains a narrative of the creation of the world and defines, through the commands of God, ethical and moral proscriptions about how one should live one's life. However, how should it be interpreted properly? If the Bible did not exist as a concrete assembly of texts, there would be no "objective" message from the past which we could relate to. However, since there exist different versions of this text, which one represents the "truth"? Which one should be considered the most valid? And what about internal contradictions in the Bible, how should they be handled? Not to speak of the different translations and how to interpret historical metaphors. That's how hermeneutics was born.

The significance of (interpretation of) written texts for the progress of science, is particularly important for the scientific status of psychoanalysis and group analysis. Are they "real" sciences, or at least evidence-based practices? The classical case stories of Freud (e.g., Fraulein Elizabeth von R, The Rat Man, Little Hans) have a special status in the history of psychoanalysis. They are written texts (objectified) that have undergone a host of later interpretations. However, the case stories themselves do not fulfil the requirements for modern research. They are stories narrated by the therapist himself, Dr. Freud. Actually, we do not know what Freud really did in these treatments. For case studies to become scientific, they must be based on interpretations of audio- or videotaped recordings which can be reinterpreted and validated or falsified by other researchers who study the same recordings ("objects"). This is particularly difficult for group analysis, also for pure pragmatic reasons. A full transcript of a group analytic session amounts to around 20 pages written text. If one should do a proper scientific study of e.g., developmental stages in group analysis and the course towards a group analytic discourse, this would need around 50 sessions, which amount to 75 hours being scrutinized, rated and interpreted, or around 1000 pages of text. To date, this has never been done. (It might be feasible in the future by help of artificial intelligence).

However, we need to go back to the topic of language as constitutive for the social world, and thereby for the self and self-consciousness. This statement needs a clarification with respect to the self as to *the distinction between the core self and the reflective self*. Let us start with the controversial issue of consciousness which is related to the mind-body/brain problem. Is consciousness a property of the brain? Yes, it is. Is it also a property of the mind? Yes. It's both, since brain and mind are closely interrelated. There is no mind without a brain. And vice versa, there is no living, functional human brain without a mind, if we by brain means an assembly of neurons at a certain stage of complexity. According to Feinberg and Barratt (2016), this level of complexity was reached around 550 million years ago with the evolution of the vertebrae species. The brains of vertebra animals were complex enough to yield a kind of map of the external world through the senses and of the internal organism through interoception and emotional awareness. These capacities were *emergent properties* of advanced neuronal complexity. To cite Eagle (2024, p. 106):

> ... biological processes are emergent phenomena that possess properties that are not possessed by the constituents of these processes. Life itself is an emergent phenomenon in so far as the chemical constituents of life do not themselves possess the property of life. It is only in the organization of these constituents that biological systems with new properties, such as homeostasis and metabolic exchange of energy, emerge. Although biological systems that emerge are subject to physio-chemical laws, new lawful regulations emerge that cannot be derived from these lower-level physio-chemical laws.
>
> Each of the above statements is applicable not only to biological, but also to psychological phenomena. In an important sense, the mind-body problem is preceded by the life-matter problem. That is, life is a property that emerges from the organization of chemical elements that alone do not have that property. And, similarly, the properties of consciousness and subjective experience emerge from the organization of physio-chemical elements that, themselves, do not have these properties.

By evolution, the agencies of sensual, interoceptive and emotional awareness were coordinated on both a neuronal and a conscious level, thus creating consciousness. Neuronal impulses "met" somewhere in the brain and through consciousness the animal could see, smell, hear and sense the external world and simultaneously regulate, trough consciousness, its position in space and its emotional responses to external events. This is *core consciousness* which gives birth to the mind and to the core self since animals are not rambling around randomly in the world but exhibit purposeful behaviour based upon subjective experiences (Northoff & Panksepp, 2008). The animal besets agency, and we should emphasize that this core self is *an embodied self* (Fuchs, 2020).

Here, we are not so interested in the senses or interoception as we are in the *emotions*. However, before we can turn to the emotions, we need to say something more about the *ontogenesis of mentalization*. We have argued that Freud and Bion were stuck at the level of words and explanatory principles of the fate of these words, which, in the best case, could be worked upon by the ego, thus transforming the meanings and implications of these words according to the reality principle. An ego was already there which could work upon the words. Fonagy et al. (2002) changed the game. It was the very development of the ego-self which was the puzzle to be solved. They maintained that in ontogenesis, the words and their meanings developed in concert with the development of the thinker. The words were already there, in the world, as elements of language. It was a question of learning the language. Thereby, the thinker would develop and thereby, the consciousness of the thinker itself, i.e., self-consciousness. *By changing the game, it became clear that the reality principle was not already there as a property of the ego. The reality principle itself had to be developed along with development of the ability to think. The reality principle became a property of a mind that beset the ability of advanced mentalizing.*

Informed by e.g., the *Theory of Mind* research, Fonagy et al. (2002) suggested that (explicit) *mentalizing proper* was a mode of thinking which most children obtained around the age of 4-5 years. The most crucial achievement was the realization by the child that other minds harboured different intentions than themselves and looked upon the world differently. Speaking with the terms of John Bowlby, they had thus achieved a *representational "model of the mind". The mind contained representations of the world, not the world itself. This is the most decisive feature of the so-called reality principle.* Fonagy et al. (2002) maintained that thinking developed according to a scheme consisting of an initial *teleological mode*, whereby cause and effect had to be observed concretely ("Aunt Mary is kind because she gave me the candy, while uncle Ben is scary since he is wearing glasses"), followed by a *psychic equivalent mode* of thinking where the way I think about the world, constitutes the world ("I feel there is a monster under the bed, therefore there is a monster under the bed"), followed by *pretend mode* thinking ("When we play, we imagine we are cowboys and Indians"), until these modes are transformed and integrated in *representational thinking* ("Grandma believes there are thieves in the garden but I know there aren't because I've checked it out" – i.e., an appropriate reality checking). It is not different words that distinguish these different modes. The differences lie at the level of sentences, with references to different kinds of logic. I.e., the different thinking modes represent *different discourse modes* which determine *the kind of meaning* which can be expressed in narrative terms. This turn to sentences, discourse modes and narration, opened the field of psychopathology to influences from the narrative turn in philosophy (Ricoeur, 1983).

Another crucial change by the approach of Fonagy et al. (2002) was the role assigned to attachment for the development of mentalizing abilities. And now we are approaching the topic of emotions. Attachment is basically a survival strategy that evolved through the advent of mammals (around 150 million years ago). Attachment rests on the evolution of the primary emotions of separation anxiety and care/love (Panksepp, 1998). The lost or hurt baby/infant emits signals of fear and separation anxiety which is perceived by the mother who comes to the rescue. Attachment did not evolve for the purpose of thinking. However, Fonagy et al. (2002) argue that for Homo Sapiens, *attachment relationship takes on a new significance for the ontogenesis of mentalizing by the individual.* Firstly, family members are the natural agents to learn the infant the language that is the key to understanding what is going on in the social world s/he is born into. Family members take these roles as representatives of the communities to which they belong. If their infants should have any chance for survival in these communities, they had to learn the language. Language is the key to understanding the rules of social life.

However, and most important, language is also key to understanding the inner world of oneself. In principle, language as a system of signs and grammar, could be learned by any kind of village teacher. However, proper learning about oneself requires attachment relationships. It requires the preverbal transactions of e.g., feeding, emotion-regulation, play and proto-conversation (Tronick, 2002; Schultz-Venrath, 2024) before it comes to the meaning of words and the social significance of speech acts. Secure attachment comes with a feeling of love and trust that paves the way for seeking (Panksepp, 1998), i.e., the urge for curious exploration of the external and internal world. And notably, the internal world is far more difficult to understand than the external. The external world can be pointed at, e.g., "this is a table" and this proposition can be verified by "everybody" and that's why the external world has a kind of "objectivity". The challenge of the subjective internal world is partly a question of words (e.g., what I experience now can be labelled anger), but it is mainly a *question of meaning of intentional mental states*. Do I *understand the emotion evoked in me* as a response to a certain social situation and do I understand the other person, the situation and myself to such a degree that I can modulate my response in a manner that suits my own interests within this particular group and society? This learning of basic mentalizing intersubjectivity requires attachment relationships. Beyond infancy, these competencies are learned and refined by a host of other interactions with peers and extended family and in kindergartens and schools. However, if the basics are not founded in early childhood, as in the most severe disturbance of disorganized attachment, the sad consequences for adult life course are terrible (Roberts et al., 2007). This brings us to the topics of emotions and the significance of mentalizing emotions.

Emotions and "symptoms" as unmentalized emotions

A great problem for psychoanalysis and group analysis has been their flawed theory of emotions and reluctance to modernize it. This sad state of affairs is connected to their epistemological theories which tend to favour metapsychology at the cost of empirical research. To state it bluntly, there is no empirical evidence for the primacy of sexual and aggressive drives from birth on. However, there are abundant evidence for the existence and gradual evolution of the following primary emotions among all mammals (including Homo sapiens): SEEKING (eager positive anticipation), FEAR, RAGE, SEXUAL LUST, SEPARATION ANXIETY, CARE/love and PLAY/joy. This is according to Jaak Panksepp (1998, 2012) and the primary emotions are here written in BOLD which was Panksepp's terminology whereby he underlined that when speaking of e.g., FEAR, it was according to the definition of FEAR as a primary emotional system. The definition of primary emotional systems was that:

- They could be identified among all mammals.
- They had an adaptive benefit as to crucial life challenges.
- They came with a typical behavioural pattern.

- They came with typical physiological reactions.
- They had a specific brain localization which implied that they might be activated by electric stimulation or manipulated biochemically.
- They were dependent on specific hormones, neuropeptides and neurotransmitters.

True, there are some disagreements among scholars on which emotions should count as "primary". E.g., Antonio Damasio (2000) would include disgust, while Silvan Tomkins (1992) would include shame. This is not any concern to us here, since the disagreements rest partly on the definition, i.e., what should count as a *primary* emotion. Panksepp and Biven (2012) regard disgust as a homeostatic affect (akin to hunger and thirst) and shame as a *social emotion*. The primary emotions should be likened to the colours on the palette of a painter. They can be mixed in all sorts of combination and take the appearance of social emotions such as shame, guilt, envy, jealousy, greed, vengefulness, hopelessness, respect, solidarity, sense of justice, reverence, etc. Social emotions presuppose self-consciousness, and a social order constituted by language.

Among the qualifications for a primary emotional system, one should notice the requirement of coming with a typical behavioural pattern, which includes the urge to hit (rage), the urge to cry (separation anxiety, sadness) and the urge to run (fear). Herein lies an alternative explanation to Freud's theory of discharge. Freud, when observing the hysterias of females in Vienna in late 1800, was correct in pointing to underlying physical and mental powers. Something urged for "discharge". What was the nature of these forces? Today, we will say it is the behavioural pressure that comes with (unmentalized) emotions. This pressure evokes FEAR in the individual. It is fear of being overwhelmed by own emotions and display to oneself and others what one REALLY feels and display one's confusion and thereby one's dependency on others which one might dislike or even hate.

This FEAR stems from unmentalized emotions which are the basic ingredients of what we label "symptoms". Human FEAR is a complex phenomenon. Partly, FEAR in itself engender FEAR, since it is unpleasant and might stimulate more FEAR, e.g., culminating in a formidable panic attack. One may FEAR to display to others that one is frightened. And one fears exposing other emotions which one wants to hide. One might also FEAR to hurt others or oneself. Ultimately, one may FEAR losing control over oneself and collapse mentally and physically. These aspects of FEAR are present to a lesser or larger degree in the diverse anxiety disorders, like panic disorder, generalized anxiety disorder, obsessive-compulsive disorder, the social and simple phobias, post-traumatic stress disorders, etc. FEAR is the common denominator, and the essence of anxiety disorders is malfunctioning of the FEAR system.

Similarly, a malfunctioning in the system for SEPARATION DISTRESS/ANXIETY is the common denominator for depressions, be it dysthymia or milder, moderate or severe major depression, or depression in bipolar disorders. SEPARATION ANXIETY comes with feelings of being abandoned, left alone, sadness, being excluded, hopelessness, pessimism, low or no energy, helplessness, joylessness, not worthy of living, suicidal ideation, etc.

The unmentalized emotions of FEAR and SEPARATION ANXIETY are the most common reasons for people seeking psychotherapy. As indicated above, they are labelled by a diversity of diagnostic categories which are basically descriptive. What it is all about is *unmentalized emotions*. So, what do we mean by that term? We mean body-mental states which plague the subject by being painful, disturbing, not wanted and basically meaningless and/or being attributed by psychic equivalent thinking to causes like God's will or punishment for evil deeds or own stupidity, etc. Emotions not being mentalized indicate that the individual, at the time of painful subjective experiences, was not able by own mental resources or by the help of benevolent others, to attribute culture-syntonic meanings to these experiences and integrate them in a self-sustaining narrative. Rather, the experiences were denied, split off or perceived as alien (Stanghellini, 2017). The experiences were part of the personal history, but not integrated as meaningful experiences in the personality and could not be narrated. Rather, the experiences, if severe enough, would coin the personality in a negative sense through disturbed development.

The more severe personality disturbances, the more unmentalized experiences in the depth of the individual, and vice versa. This view rests on the empirically validated assumption that human personality is basically constituted upon language. Our TAM theory (Karterud & Kongerslev, 2019) maintains that the basic constituents of personality are temperament (mainly primary emotions), attachment and mentalizing ability (self-consciousness). We find temperament and attachment in other mammals as well. And many of them live in smaller or larger groups. But they do not have mentalizing ability and do not live in what I have denoted as spiritual groups which are groups constituted by speech acts that define the rules, regulations, obligations and history of these groups. Human groups, to the contrary are founded upon meanings which are linguistically mediated. When emotional experiences, for different reasons, remain unmentalized, their meanings as understandable intentional subjective states get lost. The consequences precipitate as inconsistencies in the linguistic fabric of the self which is the more or less coherent system of memories, attitudes, emotions and thoughts of the person which can be more or less attuned to the prevailing Zeitgeist of the culture to which the person belongs.

But how does mentalization of emotions actually come about? Freud suggested it was on the level of neurons, Bion suggested it was on the level of words, while Fonagy et al. (2002) suggested it was on the level of *mental states*. Mentalizing mental states is a concept that might merit both Freud and Bion. Freud's neurons belong to a natural scientific discourse, and this should certainly be acknowledged. Emotions are body-mental states where a host of neurons indeed are involved. I have already mentioned how the gamma-butyric-acid system might reduce neuronal glutamate excitation and thereby calm down the *emotional system of fear* (in Freuds words "curbing wild and disorganized discharge"). And we could add how endogenic opioids can curb *mental states of separation anxiety*. Today we also know that the same effects can be achieved, e.g., curbing a panic attack by comfort, since comfort also works through hormonal and transmitter systems that involve the gamma-butyric-acid system and endogenic opioids. The act of comfort would come closest to Bion's concept of reverie. Emotion regulation is not something the baby can perform on its own. It needs another, i.e., a "container" in Bion's words. When saying "emotion regulation" in a modern discourse, we include both aspects. Yes, there is a "physical" aspect which involves neurons, as Freud rightly emphasized. And there is a mental, intersubjective aspect as well, which Bion emphasized. Somebody is comforting the person (and the feeling of being comforted makes the little person become attached to the adult).

The act of comforting happens among many mammal species and need not be linked to the realm of words. Mentalizing comes about when emotional mental states are imbued with meaning: "You should not go that far away from home", or "I shall take care of you", or "cats are not dangerous", or "yes, it hurts but it will be all right", etc. By such speech acts (and bodily comfort) the emotional arousal declines. Simultaneously, in the body/mind there develops neuronal connections between e.g., amygdala, hippocampus, hypothalamus and frontal cortex which allows for a two-way traffic, bottom-up and top-down (Panksepp & Biven, 2012). Emotional arousal stemming from the basal brain will affect thinking processes in the cortex, while thinking processes in the cortex also will influence emotional arousal. E.g., humans are capable of initiating a panic attack by way of thinking about something scary. The concept of mentalizing is used both for regulating emotional arousal and for thinking about emotional arousal. The mother mentalizes the child while comforting and saying in a gentle voice that "cats are not dangerous" and the child mentalizes (and comforts) herself by repeating to herself that "cats are not dangerous". It is not like these aspects belong to different realms of existence, like the neuronal excitations exist in a physical world (*res extensa*, according to Descartes) and the thinking processes belong to a mental world (*res cogitans*, according to Descartes). There is one world. This world can, however, be studied from different perspectives.

The major point is that emotions influence thinking processes and that thinking processes influence emotions. However, this interdependence is dimensional. There are modes of thinking that are very detached from emotions and there are emotions so strong that thinking almost becomes impossible. The latter we denote as *breakdown of mentalizing*. We may speculate about the neural correlates to breakdown of the capacity for mentalizing. It surely is connected to what we denote as *working memory* (Carruthers, 2015) where all sense modalities (including memories and emotions) are "globally broadcasted" to be thought about in concert. However, that is not the central issue for us now. Clinically, we are confronted with mentalizing breakdowns in the stories that patients tell, when they feel unable to think, when they feel compelled to do something desperate to get rid of unbearable feeling-body-states, when they refuse to think about some issues or feeling-body-states because of fear of becoming overwhelmed and "lose their mind". Clinically, we can observe how mentalizing capabilities of some individuals may collapse here and now, in the group, and most notably, we can observe how in a group the collective mentalizing ability might collapse. The collective collapse was what Bion (1961) described as "basic assumption groups". In a next paragraph I will contend that the use of the word "group" for these collective mental states is a misuse of the word. The misuse was perpetuated when Morris Nitsun (1991) coined the term "anti-group".

However, we must wait for these discussions. For now, we have reached the point where we can start the dialogue about the foundational tenets of group analysis.

The significance of communication and resonance in the work of S. H. Foulkes

In his first textbook, Introduction to group analytic psychotherapy, Foulkes (1948) argues for the "growing recognition of the basic importance of society" in psychoanalysis with reference to Erik Homburger Eriksson:

> … however, Psycho-Analysis has not yet allotted to this social side of man the same basic importance as it has to his instinctual aspect. For Freud, and for the majority of Analysts at the present day still, the social nature of man is a derivative from sexual love, or a reaction formation against incompatible destructive impulses. The infant is thought to be solipsistic, knowing nothing but his own instinctual urges, learning of the "outside" world only by a painful trial and error method.
>
> (Foulkes, 1948, p. 10)

Foulkes leans on unspecified *"progress in all the sciences"* and *"a mature, scientific point of view"* when he states (Foulkes, 1948, p.10) that:

> … the opposite is true: each individual – itself an artificial, though plausible abstraction – is basically and centrally determined, inevitable, by the world in which he lives, by the community, the group, of which he forms a part.

In this respect, Foulkes was a pioneer. He adds that *"Freud's own concepts were, of course, in this respect determined by his epoch, and if he had lived fifty years later, he would have been one of the first to correct them"*. This last statement might be a bit idealizing with respect to Freud, but for psychoanalysis as a whole it is true that it has moved in a more social, relational and intersubjective direction, although it has not adopted the theory of group analysis (Foulkes, 1948).

Foulkes then moves on (Foulkes, 1948, p. 29) to formulate his famous "Basic Law of Group Dynamics" which tries to explain why groups of "common people" might, under certain conditions, have healing capabilities:

> The deepest reason why these patients, ..., can reinforce each other's normal reactions and wear down and correct each other's neurotic reactions, is that collectively they constitute the very Norm, from which, individually they deviate.

From here on, he articulates his positive and prosocial nature of groups, in contrast to the psychoanalytic point of view at his time. With respect to therapeutic groups, he states that

> The sound part of Individuality, of character, is firmly rooted in the Group and wholly approved by it. The Group, therefore, respects and supports the emergence and free development of individuality, and Group treatment has nothing to do with making people uniformly march in step. Quite on the contrary; good Group treatment – by developing a good Group – makes both processes go hand in hand: the reinforcement of the communal ground and the freer development of the individual differences. ... Now, neurotic peculiarities, symptoms, are relieved just as much, as they can be retransformed, by Analysis, from unshareable to shareable experience, from uncommunicable experience to communicable experience. This is just what Analysis, individual or in Groups does. ... Neurotic symptoms disappear into the common pool as soon as they become communicable, and individual ingredient is now free for group-syntonic, socially acceptable, employment. That is the reason, why neurotic behavior tends to diminish in a Group and normal behavior to be supported. Does the Group know that? Not consciously, but it is forced to act in this direction by the very fact that it can only grow by what it can share, and only share by what it can communicate, and only "communicate" by what it has in "common" – e.g., in language – in common, that is, on the basis of the community at large.
>
> (Foulkes, 1948 p. 30)

The citations above convey the essence of group analysis and in fact they are quite compatible with the more modern conception of mentalizing. The crucial issue is *communication by language*. However, we should note that it is formulated in very general terms with reference to *"the Group"* (with large G), *"the individual"*, *"neurotic symptoms and behavior"*, *"the community at large"* and that the Group is attributed both mind and agency (*"does the Group know that?"*). The question now is how this looks like when it comes to concrete groups and individuals. The devil lies in the details!

One major concern is of course the role of the group analyst in facilitating the group processes whereby the "neurotic symptoms" become transformed by being verbalized. Foulkes describes the delicate balance between leading and conducting the group and its needs to find its own course of development. In particular he emphasizes a minimum of instructions and a "free-floating discussion".

> The Conductor wants to use the group as an instrument for therapy. By establishing and maintaining the group-analytic situation, he forges this instrument, and he continues refining it.

> His main function is to direct this process of group formation, to observe and to interpret events to himself and to the group.
>
> He is concerned predominantly with the present, immediate situation. He is particularly fortunate, in witnessing a dynamic display, he sees meaning in action.
>
> What needs to be interpreted is: content of communication, behavior and interpersonal relationships.
>
> The medium through which he works is communication through words and the ultimate aim is expression in articulate verbal language, which can be understood and shared by all.
>
> (Foulkes, 1948, p.135)

Furthermore:

> He must learn to play on this instrument like on an organ or an orchestra, soft pedaling some contributions, discouraging some contributions at times, he encourages others, countervoices as it were, helps to raise them from inarticulate murmurs to the dignity of articulated themes. … The better the Group Analyst, the less will his work be obvious. The more work he does in his own mind – and in particular has done through his training – the more sparing can he afford to be with active interference, and the more effective will his activity become.
>
> (Foulkes, 1948, p. 136)

In modern terms, the group analyst minds the individuals in the group analytic situation and attributes meaning to the ongoing group interaction. However, he is careful in not imposing these meanings on the group but prefer the group to articulate these meanings by itself. There is if course intricate dialectics here regarding the relation between the group and the conductor. On the one hand, the therapist is both the leader, the conductor and also a member of the group. On the other hand, Foulkes underlines that the conductor should not lead, but serve the group. The conductor *"wants to use the group as an instrument for therapy"* but he should also be an *"instrument of the group"*:

> He can be said to be the first servant of the group. He must follow the group's lead in turn. … The Conductor is directing the process, but in order to direct it he must let it develop and not disturb it by his interference. He allows himself passively to be maneuvered by the group. It is an ever-changing move over the whole scale from complete passivity to full activity. It is of fundamental importance that this is understood because it is the basic code of the Group Analyst.
>
> (Foulkes, 1948, p. 140)

However, these statements that the conductor is *"the first servant of the group"*, etc., are rather problematic since they downplay the role of the conductors "minding the group". They downplay the fact of the conductor as the creator of the group by attributing some rather mystical properties to the "group as a whole", seemingly independent of the mind of the conductor. They downplay the role of the ideal group in the mind of the group analyst, or the ideals of a group analytic discourse, by which the group analyst measures the interactions in the group, and which are operative in the depth of the mind of the group analyst, and which profoundly influence his/her meaning attribution and reflections on how to intervene (or not intervene).

From early on, the concept of the group as a whole becomes rather problematic in the writings of Foulkes:

> While having an eye on each individual member and on the effects they and their utterances have on each other, the Conductor is always observing and treating the group as a whole. The "Group as a Whole" is not a phrase, it is a living organism, as distinct from the individuals composing it. It has moods and reactions, a spirit, an atmosphere, a climate, as Klapman calls it.
>
> (Foulkes, 1948, p. 140)

These conceptualizations have haunted group analysis all the way since Foulkes articulated them in 1948. They concern the nature of human groups. What kind of beings are they? Or more generally: What is the nature of social entities? We will come back to these questions which are paramount to the understanding of mentalizing in groups.

Foulkes provided some transcripts and small vignettes and stories about a range of groups to illustrate his theoretical suggestions. None of those are particularly illuminating. Among the major shortcomings in his first treatise are the idealization of the Group as described above, and the lack of contemplation about the personalities of the group participants. Of course, one should take into consideration the professional Zeitgeist of the 1940s, when theories of personality and personality disorders where quite primitive. However, the tension between the Group and individual personality differences has been problematic all the way in the history of group analysis. Foulkes' initial solution was to add individual sessions when the cases were problematic and not being too concerned with the phenomenon of dropouts:

> The therapist should take a "rather sharp line about people who would have doubts, to make up their mind soon so that their places could be filled with other patients. As there is a preponderance of members who are strongly on the defense, he feels that that it would not be at a loss to this group if a number would drop out, so that, if possible, they could be replaced with more co-operative ones".
>
> (Foulkes, 1948, p. 74)

The second textbook of Foulkes was written in collaboration with E. J. Anthony (1957). In fact, Anthony wrote the major part. The book contained several long vignettes. However, the illustrations of Foulkes' way of working therapeutically were not transcripts. Lack of transcripts points to a serious problem from a scientific point of view. There is no text which exactly demonstrates how Foulkes (and other group analytic colleagues) worked. We are left with scarce descriptions that rely on the author's narration of what he believed was going on. That is a poor foundation for a practice which the proponents want to be based upon research.

We should be reminded here of Ricoeur's (1981) discussion of what makes hermeneutics a valid research method. We understand human phenomena more deeply when we have the verbatim script (or the videotape) available and can study it at a distance. *Objectivation and distanciation (and appropriation) are crucial concepts of text interpretation.* Only afterwards do we see what kind of drama in which we have been involved (Karterud, 1996). Then we see more clearly the depth semantics (the unconscious dynamics) of the group (as in supervision). Then we can construct a more complex and complete narrative of the group (and the interwoven personal narratives). *The matrix can be conceived as the depth structure of this narrative.*

Verbatim transcripts are also necessary to investigate the referential world of the group conductor. With what kinds of concepts, and explicit or implicit theories does the conductor interpret the transactions of the group. When Foulkes states that the main function of the conductor is to promote communication and mutual understanding among the group members, we automatically tend to believe that this was done in a phenomenological manner which resembles a modern group discourse. However, that was apparently not the case. The textbook of Foulkes and Anthony is full of references to Freudian metapsychology of incest wishes, Oedipal conflicts, sexual perversions, masochism and sadism, castration anxiety, etc. This is seen in the following description by one participant in a group with Foulkes:

> Dr F(oulkes) tried to compare me to a disgruntled child.
>
> 'So would you be disgruntled', I pointed out, 'if people dropped scorpions in your milk.'
>
> 'Well, but why must you stay a child?' he said, 'you don't seem to have liked it much when you were one.'
>
> He tried to explain to me that this possessive love was akin to the infant's desire to possess the breast completely. It was a great shock, he insisted, when infants discovered there were other objects in the world besides the breast.
>
> (Foulkes & Anthony, p. 109, 1957/1973)

Since this vignette was included in the book, this way of talking to a group member as well as the content of this interpretation, must have been inconspicuous to Foulkes and Anthony. By modern standards we raise our eyebrows. It underlines Ricoeur's thesis that interpretations by necessity "take the detour of the world". There is no pure phenomenology. Human affairs are interpreted according to something and this something in this case is Freudian metapsychology. As we shall see, this lesson from hermeneutics casts doubts upon Foulkes' universal claims of the essence of group dynamics.

These claims come with Foulkes' conception of what is a group. He envisaged a kind of linear evolutionary development of groups linked to the "fact" that

> "our species is many millions of years old" and that when modern "isolated" individuals come together in groups, they will be taken by "an absolute and irresistible need, to make contact and to re-establish the old and deeply rooted modes of group behavior". They will feel "again the compelling currents of ancient tribal feeling, it permeates them to the very core and that all their subsequent interactions are inescapably embedded in this common matrix".
>
> (Foulkes & Anthony, 1957, p. 235)

It is noteworthy that this book was revised in a second edition in 1973 and that the same formulations were repeated in his last textbook, *Group-Analytic Psychotherapy* (1975). Meanwhile, John Bowlby (1969) had published his studies on attachment. However, there is no reference to Bowlby who actually substantiated the claim of an "irresistible need to make contact". Yes, mammals form small family groups because of attachment bonds, and the most advanced mammals live in larger groups. When Foulkes envisaged human-like groups to have existed for "millions of years", he also missed the evolutionary new development of Homo Sapiens, that occurred around 2-300.000 years ago, and which gave rise to mentalizing abilities, language and thereby *spiritualized groups*.

Homo sapiens live in spiritualized groups which are *social entities*. We need to turn to John Searle (2010) to understand the essence and ontology of social entities. What kind of beings are social entities? Searle makes a strong case for the thesis that *social entities (or spiritualized groups) are constituted by speech acts:* "I hereby declare that you are a rightfully married couple", or that "Norway is declared a sovereign kingdom by this Constitution of 1905", or that there should exist something like "Group Analytic Society", or that "I, a group analyst, hereby create a therapeutic group for 8 persons which will meet at Tuesday afternoons". These social entities exist as long as their members are acknowledging the so-called *deontological powers* which are created by the *constitutive declarations*. By deontological power we mean *the rules and obligations that come with membership.* E.g., members of a therapeutic group must accept that the group consists of 9 persons, that the meeting will last for 1,5 hours and that the purpose of the group is self- and personality development. Furthermore, they must accept the right of the leader, the group analyst, to terminate membership if s/he concludes that member X is not worthy of membership. They must also accept to be seated in their chairs and to verbally express their concerns about how they are living their lives. The group exists as long as people accept the rules and obligations. If the members do not turn up to the group meetings, the group will cease to exist. The life of the group depends on definition, recognition, identification and commitment.

The explanatory power of this view is dramatically demonstrated when writing this chapter in March 2025. Because of the politics and personality of Donald Trump and the degeneration of the American Republic Party, the Western world has suffered the worst crisis since World War II. The crisis affects a wide range of institutions like WHO and the Paris milieu agreement, but most fundamentally it concerns NATO. *The constitutive declaration of NATO* contains a paragraph 5 that says that an attack on one of the member states should be regarded as an attack on all, and that all members are obliged to concerted defence actions. The Trump administration has cast doubt on its obligation to paragraph 5, and this has created shock waves through the states of Europe. Europe has been forced to reconsider its basic values, e.g., the deontological powers that come with the European values of what constitutes liberal and democratic states. These doubts and reconsiderations have affected enormous consequences for groups, institutions and societies.

The turmoil in an analytic group does not come about because of impersonal "forces" in the group matrix passes

> right through the individual members and may therefore be called a transpersonal network, comparable to a magnetic field. The individual is thought of as a nodal point in this network, as suspended in it.
>
> (Foulkes & Anthony, 1957/1973 p. 258)

These mechanical metaphors of *"network", "nodal point"* and *"magnetic field"* carry a low explanatory power. What it is all about is that people who are invited to join an analytic group come with different attachment patterns, with different emotion consciousness, with different levels of mentalizing and different motivations. In an analytic group they receive little instructions on how to proceed, and they therefore end up in fundamental problems of cooperation. What are they to cooperate with? What is the meaning behind the group and the conversation that is performed? *The deontological power of such a group is quite diffuse.* To a large extent it seems to be defined by the members themselves. What is expected of me as a member of this group? What are the rules and obligations? How do I cooperate with somebody I don't know and perhaps dislikes? What is the purpose? Self- and personality development? What is "the self"? What is personality? How is my personality? What is a good life? E.g., in a moral sense? Is it any moral in this group? How can I cooperate with somebody on issues I do not understand? Etc.

The "forces" Foulkes and Anthony speak about carry low explanatory power also since they are conceived as something else than emotional forces. Or are they? The fact is that Foulkes and Anthony inherited an outdated psychoanalytic theory of affects and at that time there was not yet any elaborated scientific theory of emotions. Accordingly, they may be excused, and we might accept the general concept of "forces" in older literature. However, this lack has persisted in group analysis up to this day. Even around 2017, influential group analytic textbooks fail to integrate a valid theory of emotions (Schlapobersky, 2016; Barwick & Wegmann, 2018).

When the concepts Foulkes and Anthony use are less theoretically speculative, they fare better, e.g., in the discussions about communication in the group where it is reasons to believe that Anthony is holding the pen. Foulkes & Anthony writes (ibid, p. 246):

> We can see then that to become conscious, to verbalize, and to communicate are integral parts of the therapeutic process. It is extremely probable that we are describing a single process, or at least various aspects and stages of a single process in using any of these terms. In a group-analytic group the force which drives members of the group to interact and communicate is encouraged and cultivated. In such a group therefore we find considerable pressure in favour of communication, in favour of understanding and being understood, in favour of increased consciousness, articulateness, and verbalization. Under this pressure and with the therapist's encouragement and skill as a translator, the inarticulate, unsharable, autistic symptoms of patients are gradually reshaped in the continual process of communication as ever more articulate formulations of problems. This process, as it unfolds, can be studied in all its variety at many levels and throws light on the essential dynamics of psychotherapy in any situation.

This formulation goes to the heart of what mentalizing is all about. In modern terms, we will say that *"the force(s) which drives members of the group to interact and communicate"* are the emotions of SEEKING (the curious exploration of the surroundings), the need for belonging (CARE) and recognition, and overcoming SEPARATION ANXIETY which trigger the need for verbal understanding in order to escape the prison of isolation and loneliness. If you want to belong to a human society, you need the language that constitutes this society. This language is a prerequisite for mental functioning, but it is not enough for the individual, since the individual may, for different reasons, harbour "inarticulate, unsharable, autistic" subjective experiences. As also mentalizing theory emphasizes, the verbal articulation of these parts of the mind is the road to mental health. This view challenges the traditional psychoanalytic concept of the unconscious.

The unconscious, unconscious processes and mentalizing

To designate unconsciousness with a noun, *the* unconscious, is problematic. It is close to designating it a "place". It becomes located somewhere in the mind, often conceived of as "below" something, e.g., below consciousness. Furthermore, it is often implied that it has some container-like nature. The unconscious contains something, mostly something highly unpleasant, even dangerous, which is the ultimate reason for the "hidden thing" to remain "locked" into the unconscious container. The thing, i.e., unpleasant/dangerous feelings and thoughts, exists in there, but yield an unpleasant urge to be expressed because of its drive nature. Drives strive for discharge. During psychoanalytic psychotherapy, the therapist may find the key to this unconscious container and lock it up by his/her way of being and above all, through his/her interpretations. This way of conceiving the unconscious implies that the hidden thing, the repressed, *is already there*, inside the container. The task of psychotherapy is to dig it out and persuade the ego to accept it.

This classical psychoanalytic conception of the unconscious is at odds with the views put forward in the above citation by Foulkes and Anthony. Their view, which is compatible with a more modern psychoanalytic view, e.g., formulated by Morris Eagle (2024), states that *the unconscious content is not already there.* Unconsciousness is more like not being able to express in words something of vital significance for one's being. There is something "inarticulate, unsharable, autistic" which cannot be communicated in words because the experiences are wordless and therefore meaningless. Furthermore, Foulkes and Anthony use the word *"increased consciousness"* which suggests that consciousness and unconsciousness are not either or phenomena. Subjective experiences might exist at the fringe of consciousness as something vague or obscure or shadowy, or as something which is there in a strange sense and bothers the person concerned, without the person being able to articulate what it is all about. Most often there are feelings of one sort or other, since feelings/emotions come with action programmes. As earlier noted, Freud conceived it that drives (which more rightly are emotions) press for discharge. A modern conception will say that emotions are bodily self-states with an inherent urge for expressing themselves. The primary emotions are motivators for actions. The overriding task for human beings is to civilize those emotional urges, which means to connect those bodily self-states to words, significance, meaning, narratives and more abstract networks of concepts. That is what mentalizing is about.

Like consciousness, mentalizing is not an all or nothing phenomenon. Like most other psychological phenomena, it is dimensional. Mentalizing is something we do, for better or worse. That's why we can measure mentalizing, (RF), on a scale ranging from -1 (very poor) to 9 (excellent). In mentalization-based treatment (MBT), originally developed for borderline patients, the current level of RF is decisive for the kind of dialogue which the therapist performs. At higher levels, the therapist might be more freely responsive. At lower levels s/he should be more considerate with regards to emotional arousal, vulnerability and degree of psychic equivalence or pretend mode thinking. The crucial factor is the therapist's availability as a dialogic partner, or co-thinker or co-mentalizer. S/he should adjust her/himself.

Basic facts about mentalizing are its linguistic nature, its reliance on neurobiological processes and that it cannot develop outside a mentalizing group. You need other mentalizing persons living in mentalizing groups to develop the capacity yourself. It is not a capacity which you "internalize" although how certain persons think and feel and express themselves might become ideals for you. It is a capacity which you develop to make sense of social and human phenomena. This capacity develops in concert with developments of a neurophysiological substrate which includes hormones until the age of early 20s when myelinization of the brain is fulfilled. As previously noted, there is a close relationship between neurophysiological developments and conceptual and narrative competence. E.g., the capacity to understand the reality and significance of different perspectives on social phenomena is acquired by most children at the age of 4-5 years. The most important mediator of this development has been proved to be the quality of the attachment relationship, e.g., how you have been minded/mentalized by attachment figures.

In the literature on mentalizing, we often read formulations like "mentalizing versus non-mentalizing modes" (Bateman et al., 2023). Such formulations should be avoided. Again – mentalizing is a dimensional phenomenon. Persons might mentalize excellently or poorly and there is no cut-off level given by nature. We should also add to the formulation of Foulkes and Anthony that in addition to "inarticulate, unshareable and autistic" parts of the mind, there are contents of the mind which are poorly mentalized in the sense that the content is poorly thought through and avoided because of its psychic equivalence nature combined with shame, guilt or other feared emotions. In the outskirts of consciousness, for some people, thinking certain narratives might feel like doing them.

In essence, mentalizing is the capacity to think about mental states and this capacity can be more or less developed or sophisticated. It will never be "fully developed" since there is no endpoint here. Persons will struggle to understand themselves, other people and the ever-changing world from the cradle to the grave. Do we also perform unconscious mentalizing? As noted, we should be cautious with the concept of THE UNCONSCIOUS, e.g., as a place where some strange ideation can take place. If so, how can we then understand dreams? Freud's work on dreams (1900) was a landmark event in the evolution of psychoanalysis. Here he formulates his decisive theory of the manifest versus the latent content of the dream. The latent content belongs to the unconscious and is ruled by other principles than the reality principle of the ego. However, by definition, we cannot speak by certainty of what is going on in THE unconscious and what kind of principles that reign there. By definition, our hypotheses are kind of speculations. Is any mentalization going on there? Or is mentalizing, by definition, something which goes on in e.g., working memory? If one accepts this last proposition, one should *change focus from THE unconscious to unconscious processes.* There are a lot of causes and reasons for our behaviour which we are unaware of, or have a poor understanding of, or outright deny. Above all, this is about our attitudes, as part of our personality. They operate silently, in the background, as "the way we are".

In a group, "the way we are" will become apparent through behaviour, narratives and speech acts. Other group members will react and say things like "you are too modest", "you should be more self-assertive", "you are so emotional", "you are so dominant", "you are too submissive", "you talk too much", "you should speak more", "you are arrogant", "you are too envious", "you are too kind", "actually you are passive-aggressive", "you are so self-derogatory", "I get provoked by your helplessness", etc. For some people, this might come as a surprise. They "don't see it". However, other people "see it" and they have opinions about the negative consequences these attitudes have for you. In group-analytic literature one often sees the expression that the group is likened to a "hall of mirrors". There you might "see" aspects of yourself of which you were not aware.

This will be the most common understanding of unconsciousness in group analysis. It refers to attitudes you are not or poorly aware of. These attitudes are not located as propositions in a kind of space which we can label THE unconscious and which are thought about "in the unconscious". The attitudes have a lot of sources, like temperamental dispositions (primary emotions), attachment experiences, other crucial experiences in schools and among peers and social media, traumas, habits, mimesis, coincidences, bad luck, etc. To be more aware of and being able to think about those attitudes which compose the fabric of yourself, you need to see yourself more "from the outside". It "takes a detour of the world", as Ricoeur says. It takes a group. By that, you will be more able to differentiate between constructive and prosocial parts of yourself and the more dysfunctional attitudes and ways of thinking and relating. Dialectical behaviour therapy talks about emotion dysregulation, while cognitive therapy talks about dysfunctional maladaptive cognitive schemas. In reality it is often both, interwoven in the fabric of personality. In a therapeutic group, these related aspects will become visible.

A modern psychoanalytic view on consciousness and unconsciousness (Eagle, 2024) highlights the importance of *communication*. What is unconscious cannot be communicated in words by the protagonist. However, it is partly communicated "under the words" or "between the lines", as a subtext, and by attitudes, absences and behaviour (Gullestad & Killingmo, 2019). Therefore, s/he needs a skilful and receptive dialogue partner. The good news about group analysis is that transcendental communication can take place also in groups, conveyed by trained and friendly peers. I write "trained" because group members become trained as *competent* group members through their experiences in good analytic groups. There is nothing magic in groups in and by themselves. They might be boring, oppressive, rigid, scapegoating, etc. It is the theory and practice of the group analyst that enables the group to develop the rare type of culture that can be denoted as "group-analytic", whereby the group members learn to practice a certain type of communication. And this type of collective communication is a product of historical developments in the Western culture. It could not have been created in e.g., Muslim cultures during the midst of the 20th Century, since group analysis presupposes the ideals and attitudes of autonomy and freedom, free and open communication/speech and lack of taboos, be they religious or about women's rights or gender identity.

The Western Zeitgeist which gave birth to group analysis is well described by Taylor (1989) in his *Sources of the Self. The Making of Modern Identity.* Modern identity, with all its assets and limitations, is a product of a long history of ideas and battles for power and freedom. Most significant is the process of secularization. Today we have difficulties in imagining the fundamental impact religion used to have for people, groups and societies as organizer of believes about the nature of things (Taylor, 2007). Secularization implied a totally different way of grounding individual and group existence. Above all, morality had to find a new justification. How can I justify what is good and morally right for me compared to the needs of others as individuals or representatives of group values? Western civilization has gone far in the direction of declaring the rights of the individual. This is accompanied by an attitude of *inwardness* and *autonomy*. Instead of contemplating what might be the will of God, modern identity is linked to a search for what is good for ME. I must look *inside myself*. And that might be quite confusing. Where and by what do I find the grounding for this autonomy? Thereby the question of THE SELF becomes paramount. The striving for a Western identity has also implied contradictions between an attitude of rationality and belief in science and technology on the one hand, and romanticism on the other hand. *Romanticism* implied that vital sources of the self were to be found in sentiments and emotions which were linked to the nature of man in harmony with the nature of the universe and that these emotions required to be *expressed*. A vital life, a life worth of living required a kind of inwardness that opened for the natural sources of life, regardless of modern technology. Furthermore, a modern Western identity implied an enhanced emphasis on *ordinary life*. The major concern of most modern westerns is not any longer how to live in accordance with religious rules and restrictions, but how to organize, contemplate and negotiate the demands of ordinary daily life with families, friends and colleagues in a society governed by liberal democratic rules and values.

According to Habermas (1984), the morality of such a society should be grounded in an *ethics of communication*. Freedom depends on the quality of communication within the society. Above all, according to Habermas, it should be free of dominion ("herrshaft-frei"). It was in the same period that Grice (1989) formulated his principles for a rational discourse. We have already noted how the principles of Rice influenced Mary Main and coworkers when they constructed the *Adult Attachment Interview* which was the main source of inspiration for Peter Fonagy and coworkers when they constructed the manual for assessment of Reflective Functioning (mentalizing). This manual is essentially a manual for assessing *the quality of a person's deliberations about him/herself*. What we can see here is a fruitful interaction between philosophy and psychology. Philosophy explores general ontological questions, like "what is the nature of man?". In the postwar period we see a philosophical turn to linguistics, i.e. language *constitutes* the essence of being human. We communicate by *speech acts*. And we do all sort of things by speech acts, e.g., create social realities like groups and institutions. We even create (human and self-reflective) consciousness by speech acts. However, philosophy was not preoccupied with individual differences, which became the topic for personality psychology. Psychology, as an empirical discipline, must go beyond the general ontological question about what the nature of man is, to the question of what the nature of an individual human being is. By this turn, psychology encounters individual differences. While philosophers like Habermas were concerned with societal restrictions upon free and open communication, psychoanalysts could observe *the restrictions that came from the inner world of the individuals*, i.e. from the depths of their personality. However, there was a dialectic here. The external and the internal sources of oppression influenced each other. Groups and individuals should be liberated in concert. That was the radical thesis of Foulkes.

Some later developments in group analytic theory

We have seen how the "radical Foulkes" opened for communication in his group analytic theory but above all in his therapeutic practice in a way compatible with the modern theory of mentalizing. However, he never formulated anything close to a conception of human individuals and groups being *constituted* by language. His theory of Groups was a strange mixture of romantic and mechanical conceptualizations. Groups were basically good but haunted by powerful forces. How have these contradictions been handled by later literature?

In my previous book, *Group Analysis. A Modern Synthesis*, I describe some important post-Foulkesian trends. The efforts of Malcolm Pines (1990, 1996a, 1996b) (and partly by Dennis Brown) to import concepts, theories and practices from American self-psychology did not leave many traces. More important were the efforts by Nitsun (1996) to integrate the theories of Klein and Bion. In my opinion, this was a blind alley. "Destructive forces in groups" came to be understood by metapsychology through the concept of an "anti-group" rather than by modern theories of personality pathology and their interpersonal and collective consequences.

However, for our present purpose, let us go straight to the most recent and textbook-like volume by Schlapobersky (2016) *From the Couch to the Circle. Group-Analytic Psychotherapy in Practice.* The book is not very well organized, but the content is mainly an expansion of Foulkes' major contribution which was about communication in groups. In this sense it is truly "Foulkesian". And it is clinical, as Schlapobersky writes (2016, p. 7):

> Much of the contemporary literature in group analysis favours metapsychology and theory at the expense of key practical questions that our trainees face at the workplace.

Schlapobersky's work is truly an expansion of Foulkes, and he writes (2016, p. 16) that

> Foulkes's own writing leaves questions of therapeutic method – of how to practice – strangely incomplete.

In other words, it was not that Foulkes was "wrong" on some issues, but that he was "incomplete".

Schlapobersky condenses his contribution to 12 *"basic principles in group-analytic psychotherapy"* which include highly relevant themes such as prerequisites for group and personal development, about structure, process and content of therapeutic groups, about the diverse roles of the conductor, about process dynamics, the group as an auxiliary ego, the relational field, the vicissitudes of intersubjective validation, and above all *on monologue, dialogue and discourse* in groups. The last themes, on monologue, dialogue and discourse, are original contributions by Schlapobersky and here he comes closest to the conception of the human self being constituted by language, without stating it explicitly.

Schlapobersky maintains the tradition of highlighting the importance of *free-floating discussion* in analytic groups. This is an issue of outmost importance both theoretically and clinically. When discussing this theme, we should remember that Schlapobersky's clinical practice was of a "classical" London group-analytic style with twice-a-week groups and treatment durations of e.g., 5–10 years. Within this context, Schlapobersky find it meaningful to compare this ideal of free-floating discussion to the psychoanalytic forerunner, that of free associations, as a means to get access to the unconscious. However, the principle of free associations is a psychoanalytic dogma founded in early versions of psychoanalysis. It is based upon a solipsistic conception of the mind/self and a conception of the unconscious as already containing difficult, but organized thoughts. By free associations the analyst might get access to the unconscious content by bypassing the defences. That is not how we look upon it today. Modern psychoanalysis is more and more relational and based upon dialogues more than free associations (Eagle, 2024). It is the quality of the dialogue that counts. The silent and contemplating psychoanalyst who delivers his/her wise interpretations is a ghost from the past. This development makes the topic even more difficult and complex. It is not a matter of free associations or not, or free-floating group discussions or not. It is a question of degrees, of more or less, and what we mean with these expressions "free" and "free-floating".

Schlapobersky has several good clinical illustrations in his book (e.g., Schlapobersky, 2016, pp 117–130) which give rich substance to the claim of liberating individual inhibitions and promoting personal growth, from alienating monologues through mutually engaging dialogues to a kind of group discourse that involves all participants. The processes are simultaneously relational and semantic. People engage with each other while they expand on their understanding of self and others. In these illustrations, the conductor plays a mainly facilitating role in commenting in a constructive manner on the communicational processes in the group. E.g., after a while the conductor asks the monologue patient "who he is talking to" (Schlapobersky, 2016, p. 117). What Schlapobersky describes is increased quality of the way patients talk and relate to each other, and he uses the expression "in a mature group at this stage" (Schlapobersky, 2016, p.124). The discourse becomes rich, complex, relevant and important for individuals and the group as a whole. He distinguishes between structure, process and content and writes (Schlapobersky, 2016, p. 280):

> Differentiation between the dimensions of structure, process and content is notional. A group's content will not be therapeutically productive unless it is set in context by productive work in the other two dimensions. Metaphors only become therapeutically mutative when the warp and the weave – the structure and the process – are in place. Free-floating discussion develops through interplay between narrative and drama, story and exchange, reconstruction and encounter.

> Discourse describes the communication of thought by speech, the exchange between someone speaking, someone listening, and something listened to, the relationship between narrator, listener and story. The language of a group is a form of behaviour in the group, a way of referring to experience in and beyond the group and a way of transforming experience in and beyond the group. The use of discourse theory to explore free-floating discussion can give clinical depth … As the conductor reviews the group's dynamics, they will gain purchase on the process by asking themselves the following questions: Who is speaking? To whom are they speaking? What are they speaking about – what is the message? What is not being said? The two additional questions introduced here are: Should the conductor intervene in any of these areas? If so, then on what terms?

Schlapobersky gives the conductor the following discourse recommendations (Foulkes, 1948, p. 282):

Conductor's challenge	*Therapeutic purpose*
Promote narrative and narrative encounter.	*Foster interaction and intersection between people's stories (1) so people can find their own voice and (2) so they can discover their position in relation to one another.*
Develop a sense of enquiry into the group's narrative and thematic development.	*The spirit of enquiry planted in the group by the conductor needs to grow amongst its members. Thematic and narrative analysis will come to be undertaken by all the group's members.*
Crystallise thematic development with group-as-a-whole observations.	*Bridge different people's contributions with linking observations, especially when this does not happen by itself.*
Work with the modalities of time and space generated by the group and bring them round to the dynamic present.	*Foster systematic exploration of members' past and present, inside and beyond the group, and then bring this into the dynamic present.*
Listen to the voice of the symbol and educate the group's members in how they too can hear it.	*The group's process is explored for the metaphors it generates, and this in turn allows its metaphors to have purchase on the process. What is looked for in the movement between content and process is the discovery of meaning in the implicate order of experience.*

The above citations display Schlapobersky at his best. The content is free of metapsychological jargon. It's about people, language, discourse and the effort to understand each other in the performance of a difficult task (mutual understanding of self and others). The conductor takes a leading role in promoting a certain type of discourse. He does not impose discourse rules to the group but tries to encourage a certain way of thinking and relating. This is far from the starting point of group analysis which attributed many of these capabilities to a strange notion about "the group itself". However, Schlapobersky himself hesitates to go into a theoretical discussion with Foulkes about the sources of this peculiar group discourse which we denote as group analytic. We will discuss that in the next paragraph.

I have praised Schlapobersky for his elaborations on monologues, dialogues and discourse in group analysis and *thereby strengthening the linguistic and communicative foundation of group analysis.* Thereby, he also contributes to a deeper understanding of mentalizing. The theory of mentalizing is traditionally linked to a two-person psychology. The prototype is the parent/mother who minds the baby/child and thereby provides linguistic meaning to the emotional experiences of the child who organizes his/her personal experiences around this meaning. Sometimes, this process will of course be a kind of faulty mirroring that alienates the child, but that is not what concerns us most now. This meaning formation can be understood as "the colossal forces from outside" which Foulkes was so concerned about when he emphasized that forces that affected the individual was not merely something from the inside, from the drive pressure of the id, but had a social origin. How the mother experience and thinks about her child are dependent on a wide range of factors. Peter Fonagy and coworkers (1991) has shown that one important source is the mother's own attachment pattern. However, that does not explain everything. The way the parent/mother thinks and feels is deeply influenced by the culture of her family, neighbourhood, friends, occupation, economy and social class. Furthermore, there is a well-known strong correlation between attachment patterns and socio-economic conditions. E.g., the poorer socio-economic conditions (with low income, unemployment, criminality, drug abuse, high divorce rates, child neglect and abuse), the more insecure attachment pattern of the children (Roberts et al., 2007). The mentalizing ability of the caregiver is thus deeply influenced by the ability to think and reflect and maintain coherence around human values by the surrounds. It illustrates how mentalizing is not confined to a two-person process of meaning-formation and thus supports Foulkes thesis of the influence of "social forces". Mentalizing belongs to the sphere of narratives which derive their meanings from a higher level of discourse. The way meaning-formation happens in groups is well described by Schlapobersky (and other group analytic authors). Above all, it's not a linear process. We cannot predict where (when and by whom) there will occur a genuine process of mutual understanding that have the power to transcend previously more rigid and restricted ways of thinking, feeling and relating. The contributions of group analysis lie in the descriptions of group resonance, location, condensation, translation and interpretation (Foulkes & Anthony, 1957; Schlapobersky, 2016). The overriding message is that the mentalizing ability of the individual to a large degree is dependent on the mentalizing ability of the collective/group of which s/he is a member. The group conductor should therefore invest most of his energy and skills in the development of the group's ability to perform a high-quality collective group discourse. By that means, the individual might find him/herself in a mentalizing milieu with more opportunities and challenges than in most individual therapies.

The "forces" Foulkes spoke about are emotions. Emotions are necessary for things to matter. When the prototype parent/mother "minds" her baby/child it is because something matters, whether it is because of love/care, play, anger, fear, seeking, sexual arousal or seeking (or social emotions like shame, guilt, envy, pride, etc.). This minding may be more or less appropriate for what is going on (emotional state) in the mind of the child. Faulty mentalized, or unmentalized, significant mental states might leave scars that impact personality development and sooner and later will make themselves known as (mental/bodily) symptoms. Symptoms are almost by definition unmentalized emotions. E.g., unmentalized separation anxiety will appear as some kind of depression and unmentalized fear will appear as some kind of anxiety disorder. It is disappointing, therefore, that Schlapobersky perpetuates the group-analytic tradition of neglecting the issues of personality and emotions. In that sense, his 2016 book is strangely old-fashioned. There is almost no dialogue with the personality disorder literature, as if this belongs to an alien universe. And the topic of emotions is almost absent, except for the stories told in the many clinical vignettes. Emotions are of course covered in these stories, often very strong emotions, but there is no reference to any theory of emotions, nor to theories of personality and emotions, and nothing about the conductor in this respect, whether s/he works as to enhance emotion consciousness.

What we encounter then, in this modern textbook of group analysis, is a progressive elaboration of communication and discourse in therapeutic groups alongside with a sound distance to metapsychological speculations while at the same time a reluctance to enter into dialogue with modern empirical discourse on emotions and personality problems.

A couple of years later, in 2018, two younger group analytic colleagues, Nick Barwick and Martin Weegmann, published another textbook-like volume, *Group Therapy. A Group-Analytic Approach.* Was this younger generation able to follow up and expand on Schlapobersky's emphasis on communication and discourse and integrate as well modern theories of emotions and personality? Not to any significant degree. They do a clever update on traditional Foulkesian theory and practice, but it lacks a critical historical perspective, including challenges for the future. It is a progress that mentalizing and MBT is mentioned although in a rather cursory manner. The shortcomings are painfully demonstrated in an account by Nick Barwick about his experiences with a group in an outpatient psychotherapy department of a psychiatric hospital. Here, group analysis hits the wall of modern realities in the National Health Services. There is a stark contrast to stories told by Schlapobersky from the carefully organized twice-a-week group in a London private practice. Barwick struggles with a group composed of patients who display severe personality problems. For some reasons or other, they were not properly diagnosed:

> I am describing here some of the characteristics of narcissistic and borderline personalities. They were also the characteristics of several members of my group.
>
> (Barwick & Weegman, 2018, p. 141)

It is a pity that Barwick does not describe the essence of narcissism and borderline in modern terms but devote several passages to referring and elaborating upon the notion of "psychic skin" by Esther Bick (1968/1988). There is nothing wrong with Esther Bick, but there is something wrong with an account in 2018 of group dynamics with borderline patients that prefer the metaphor of "psychic skin" to an empirically based discourse on borderline dynamics. The clinical course of Barwick's group is not surprising. It is filled with distrust, suicidal threats and gestures, "distressing rows and precipitous departures" (Bick 1968/1988, p. 156) although it slowly develops a bit more mutual trust and cohesion. The problem with this account is that it lacks references to a large theoretical and clinical literature that previously has experimented with, described and researched dynamic group psychotherapy with this population (summarised in Karterud, 2015, 2023). This literature has come up with a range of structural and technical suggestions on how to avoid such miserable group dynamics as Barwick describes. The sad story is that there has been too little dialogue between group analytic circles and other approaches that has started to compete with the hegemony of group analysis (Karterud et al., 2024). We will return to this problem after having finished our discussion about the nature of groups.

What is a group? We can do without a group mind but need a group matrix. Social ontology and a critique of Bion's and Nitsun's use of the concept "group"

Schlapobersky (2016, p. 125) accepts Foulkes' rather vague theory about a group matrix and even a group mind. In a short paragraph discussing the interplay between the relational and semantic field of the group, he cites Foulkes:

> It becomes easier to understand our claim that the group associates, responds and reacts as a whole. The group as it were avails itself now of one speaker, now of another, but it is always the transpersonal network which is sensitized and gives utterances, or responds. In this sense we can postulate the existence of a group 'mind' in the same way as we postulate the existence of an individual mind.
>
> (Foulkes, 1964, p. 118)

And Schlapobersky adds (2016, p. 125):

> The group 'mind' can now be understood as the composite of its semantic and relational elements.

The above sentence by Schlapobersky is hardly meaningful. How can the "group mind" now be understood as "the composite of its semantic and relational elements"? What does that mean? In what sense? And what about the acceptance of Foulkes claim that "we postulate the existence of an individual mind" in the same manner as we "postulate the existence of a group mind"? The individual mind is not a "postulate", it is a biological and social fact. We can do research on it and map its most important constituents, e.g., the hippocampus, amygdala and the orbitofrontal cortex and their interconnecting neuronal networks. However, we can have divergent opinions about the nature of this mind, e.g., how much it is influenced by interpersonal and group processes. Compared to the notion of an individual mind, the notion of a group mind is vastly speculative and without support in any Western academic circles outside some minor group analytic milieus. A vague concept of a group mind was part of (German) romantic ideation in the 18th century and was scandalized by the Nazi movement in the 1920-1930s. Today we would rather talk about group and national mentalities, e.g., when we say the French in some respects are different from the Germans.

Why do group-analytic circles continue with this discourse about a group mind and the group matrix as "a network of forces that penetrate the individual to its innermost core"? Part of the explanation, I believe, is a *collective idealization* of Foulkes (Karterud, 2000). E.g., it is stated in the declaration of European Group Analytic Training Institutions Network (EGATIN) that it is an international training institution for "*Foulkesian group psychotherapy*". In contrast, most psychoanalytic institutes do not state that they are training institutions for "Freudian psychoanalysis". They train professionals in psychoanalysis. Secondly, there is always an established habit in ways of thinking and expressing oneself that is part of a social practice that confirms the identity of the social institution in question. "That's the way we speak in this group/region/country". Thirdly, the matrix concept has been regarded as almost sacred, as one of the cornerstones of group-analytic theory. If you touch that, what will then remain?

True, there is something supra-individual which group analysis holds on to, and which is important to discuss. It is a social fact that people affect each other to strong degrees in groups. How can we conceptualize that without resorting to the mechanical metaphors of the traditional matrix concept? I will suggest a redefinition of the terms. But how should we proceed? Do we get any help from the theory of mentalizing? One option is to go back to phenomenology and hermeneutics. E.g., what are the subjective experiences we try to explain? And how are these affected by "forces"? In my book *Group Analysis. A Modern Synthesis* (2023) I argue at length for the necessity of a conception of the self along the philosophical lines of

Paul Ricoeur and the psychological lines of Heinz Kohut. Furthermore, I follow Kohut in his reflections about the group self. The subjective side of the self is I and ME, while the subjective side of the group self is WE and US.

This subjective experience of I/me fluctuates according to my mental state which is impacted by the situation in which I find myself. In our times we describe these mental states with reference to one's personality structure which is composed of one's temperamental dispositions (mainly emotional), one's attachment strategies, one's core self-identity and one's capacity for mentalization (self-reflection/consciousness). There is robust research evidence behind these conceptualizations (Karterud & Kongerslev, 2019, 2021). The group-analytic theory about the tripartite matrix (Nitzgen, 2024) contains a concept of a "personal matrix" which is vaguely defined (Karterud et al., 2019). This vague concept should definitely be modernized. Whatever fluctuations in my mental state that may occur, they occur to ME. The me stems from my core identity, my feeling of selfhood.

In the same way, the subjective feeling of us, of being a we, is a fluctuating experience, depending on what happens in the group. However, like the subjective experience of I/me, it is most often not chaotic or random. It depends on a range of phenomena. Some of them inside each group member, like their attachment patterns, but above all it's an intersubjective, or transsubjective, experience. We-ness in a group is a feeling of connectedness around a common project or purpose. We-ness corresponds to selfhood. It fuels an experience of bonding and mutual identification. It is based upon the primary emotions of CARE/love, a reduction of FEAR and SEPARATION ANXIETY and opens for renewed SEEKING and mutual PLAY. It fuels *collective intentionality* and solidarity. We cooperate and explore the world together. We trust each other and support each other. Thereby, in an analytic group we can assist each other for exploration of painful depths of the individual's mind. This subjective feeling of we-ness is not necessarily experienced in the same way by all participants, since group members are different with respect to their attachment patterns and emotion consciousness. Furthermore, they are different with respect to their ability to grasp the meaning and significance of what is going on in the group (different levels and profiles of mentalizing). But clinicians do observe again and again how even detached group members become affected and participate constructively in moving sequences in groups which are ruled by a group analytic discourse as Schlapobersky defines it.

In discussing this issue about we-ness, we should remember the vast empirical literature on *group cohesion*. There is abundant evidence for the members' subjective experiences of group cohesion as being the most important factor for individual development and symptom relief (Burlingame et al., 2018). Group cohesion measures the degree to which a person agrees with the purpose of the group, its way of working and how s/he bonds with the therapist and the other group members.

When confronted with such truly group phenomena which exist on a higher "level" than the individual or the dyad, we realize that we need concepts that can clarify the nature of these higher-level phenomena. Which concepts are most useful and how can they be defined? As noted before, I have suggested the concept of the group self. The great advantage with that concept is that is takes care of the phenomenon of we-ness and implicitly of group identity. We are gathered and cooperate for a purpose. The ideals and ambitions of the group are embedded in this foundation and group members take on different roles in the efforts of the group to realize its goals. They act on behalf of a supraordinate project.

But what about the group mind? If something should earn the label of being the group mind, the foremost candidate might be the conductor. He is both a member of the group, its leader and the conductor. And the group is his "baby". S/he initiated it, and s/he has seen it grow up. S/he is concerned about its life and want it to survive and flourish. S/he mentalizes the group by contemplating about what is going on and how to assist it in the best possible way. As Foulkes said, s/he is the servant of the group. As well as its parent, I would add. Importantly, as a good parent, this "group mind" reflects about the group between its meetings. When I'm doing individual psychotherapy, I always ask myself how did last session impact upon the patient. What did it set in motion? With that curiosity in mind, I always start individual sessions by the question "where should we start?", implying that I am interested in what has been going on in the client's mind and what has concerned him/her the most. In the same way, I always start an analytic group with the same question. "Where should we start?" The question is not mere rhetoric. It springs out of an *engaged curiosity*. It is contrary to the attitude of Bion who recommended an analyst stance "without memory and desire" (Bion, 1967). Bion's ideal analyst should rid him/herself of previous thoughts, emotions and knowledge about the patients to become the ideal container where true "reverie" could take place, i.e., converting beta-elements to alfa-elements that could be thought about. As I have explained earlier in this chapter, this is not how mentalizing theory goes. Mentalizing is not about words. It is about meaning and that implies narratives. When I am thinking about the group between sessions, I am thinking about who said what to whom and how did the other members respond and how possibly did that affect the group as a whole and what did it possible set in motion? Since this last encounter, what has been going on in the minds of the group members? And how has that affected their experience of we-ness, alliance, bond, purpose and ability to cooperate on mentalizing deep existential concerns? I am not neutral about it. I am prepared for more pain and anger and grief, but I hope that the group has gained more collective competence in dealing with these emotions. I do also believe that if I do not think in this way, I will do a bad service for the group, i.e., if I stop being a dialogue partner for the group and rely on some unknown "forces in the matrix" or some mysterious process of "reverie".

However, even how significant the conductor might be, he is obviously not the total group mind. He works in concert with the other group members. Together they realize something which is embedded in the depth of the group. It is the notion of some specific purpose which is absent in the Foulkesian concept of the group mind. He writes about an abstract Group that wants to realise something. But not what this something *is*. As if groups can be abstracted from their purpose. The concept of the group self, however, comes with certain ambitions and ideals that are historically situated. E.g., an analytic group conductor cannot be understood as an abstraction. When s/he initiates a certain analytic group, s/he does not operate in pure private subjectivity. S/he enacts a certain historical tradition. S/he becomes a spokesperson for the ambitions and ideals that are embedded in the group analytic traditions, i.e. its group self (Karterud, 2023).

With respect to group self and we-ness, let's take another detour by Donald Trump. I find myself as a Norwegian in a Western world that is shattered by his (and his coworker's) behaviour. Trump delivers continuous attacks on Western we-ness, and his behaviour illuminates what group cohesion and we-ness is all about. As I have noted earlier, it is based upon constitutive declarations that come with deontological power. If one should furnish the matrix concept with new meaning, I believe that's the closest we come on its essence. The matrix of the Western world has consisted of declarations of mutual values, support and cooperation on a wide range of vital issues such as defence (NATO), health (WHO), work regulations (WTO), milieu (Paris declaration), tariff systems, foreign aid, values such as a shared understanding of what a liberal democracy is all about, etc. – all being maintained by a certain code of diplomatic conduct. Mutual international agreements of these kinds have been the very foundation (matrix) of the Western world.

These constitutions are not "unconscious". They have been there silently in the background as *silent premises for the Western feeling of we-ness*. When the most important partner in this cooperation declares that former constitutive declarations are not valid any longer, and to the contrary starts to behave in a threatening manner, it affects everybody. If a concept of the matrix should be meaningful, it should contribute to a profound understanding of phenomena as described above. It is hard to see how such a concept can do without a theory of social institutions being constituted by speech acts. That brings matrix closer to the concept of the group self which definitely is constituted by acts of speech. The group self-concept also takes care of the agentic aspect of groups, which Foulkes attributed to a Group Mind. Yes, we need some concepts which can be useful for the fact that groups, as such, have agendas. They are constructed for certain purposes. But we should not attribute such agendas to an abstract romantic idea about a Group Mind. This idea should be abandoned.

We are left with the concepts of matrix and group self. These concepts should be linked to the question: "what is a group?". Earlier in this chapter, I have referred to John Searle and his theory of social ontology which I find convincing. Social entities are different from material entities. A mountain, or the earth for that case, exist independent of our opinions about it. Social entities do not. A dollar bill counts as money because we (i.e., the banking system) believes in it. If US goes bankrupt, or changes to crypto, the dollar bill becomes worthless. It does not count as money any longer but continues to be a piece of paper. Social entities are thus created by constitutive speech acts. We declare something to be. Groups belongs to this category. By "groups" we here mean something more than an occasional assembly of people. Groups are organized around a purpose. Be it maintenance of a family, a tribe, a football club, a scientific committee or a therapeutic group. We also need to remember the difference between e.g., a chimpanzee tribe and a human group. Human groups are organized according to verbally expressed purposes.

This definition of what a (human) group is, is contrary to the use of "group" in the discourse of e.g., Bion (1961) and Nitsun (1996). Bion writes about "basic-assumption groups" (BA-groups) and Nitsun about "anti-group". However, strictly speaking a BA-group (or an anti-group) is not a group. It is a collective mental state which groups sometimes can be dominated by, like states of fear, helplessness, guilt, sexual desire, joy, eager anticipation, etc. Most often it is not even the case that "the group" is dominated by these emotions, but that it concerns a powerful majority or "elite" of the group who act as if they are the rightful spokespersons of the group. Similarly, we do not speak about an angry-person or an anti-person, but about persons who are in a state of anger or persons who are in a state of antagonism. Sometimes Bion and Nitsun also speaks of BA-groups and anti-groups as being groups in states of collective emotions but often they speak of BA-groups and anti-groups as if they are entities in their own right, acting on the members from behind so to speak and forcing them to act in certain ways. In such instances the noun "group" is taken literally, and the literature is replete with examples of such reification of the concepts BA-groups and anti-group. The "group" is conceived as an object that attacks the group members from within. This way of resonating conveys confusion about the nature of groups.

The matrix has traditionally been understood as a "web" which "channels communication". "Forces" in the group are transported through this web, and they "penetrate" the individuals who are conceived as "nods in this web" to their innermost core. How can we translate this discourse to understandable language? Firstly, a web indicates a structure. Somebody, i.e., the group members, are connected through this web. This connectedness becomes established out of something. It is not at random, and it does not come out of the blue. It is designed and planned to last for a certain time. Although, some matrices are thought of existing forever, such as the Catholic Church or an area called Europe or the European Union. On the other side, there are occasional meetings of somebody, lasting for some short moments, like people assembling in the street because of a traffic accident. These last encounters are not groups in an institutional sense. Institutional groups have a certain duration. You become member of something, and you cooperate with something.

The dynamic matrix is the established way of cooperation in a group which may be more or less constructive. Once established, the reason for the prevailing group norms may be forgotten. New members may take them as "natural". "That is simply how it is". They don't experience them as so-called "group solutions" to use the term of Dorothy Whitaker (1981), e.g., that some group norms are compromises due to older group controversies. Some group norms have obvious defensive purposes and the group analytic literature about group matrix has traditionally been concerned with the impact of unprocessed collective traumas (Hopper, 2014) where certain individuals and subgroups carry the burden of being victims for events in the past which the larger group tends to deny. However, we should remember that collective traumas need not be the rule in the history of groups and societies. For well-functioning groups and societies, like the Scandinavian nations, the rule is that prosocial norms have prevailed and made the collective institutions reasonably well equipped to deal with the inevitable conflicts that communal life contains.

Concerning the foundation matrix, you have not chosen it. You have been born into it, and it is therefore deeply ingrained in you. You owe the foundation matrix the very capacity to think (mentalize) as well as the specific language you are born into, and the habits and characteristic attitudes which are part of the identity of your culture. E.g., as a Norwegian, I speak the Norwegian language and consider Denmark and Sweden to be "sibling" nations because of similar language and history. I am ingrained in attitudes such as a high degree of mutual trust, that the bureaucracy works for my interest and that it therefore is quite OK to pay taxes, that I support liberal democratic and secular values, that I support human rights and equality and held the value of autonomy high. I want the freedom to realize my life project according to my personal values and preferences. One should note that *such attitudes* are to be reckoned to belong the foundation matrix, which has been somewhat overlooked in group analytic literature. The foundation matrix should also reflect differences between nations and civilizations. E.g., that there are crucial differences between European and Muslim cultures. History, or more precisely, historical precipitates or consequences are therefore part of the foundation matrix, as outlined by Norbert Elias (1978, 1982) in his monumental work on Civilization (and The Germans, Elias 1996).

Therefore, the foundation matrix is created in principle in the same way as the dynamic matrix, i.e., through constitutive speech acts which set in motion deontological powers that shape history. E.g., Norway as a nation (institutionalized group) owes much of its foundation to the Country Law of 1274, as formulated by the king Magnus "Lawmaker" and accepted by regional landlords throughout the country. This law formulated the rules and obligations that should count for citizens of the kingdom of Norway. E.g., how disputes should be settled, how a murder should be handled, how peasants should cooperate about road construction and maintenance, how much and how taxes should be paid, the rights of women, rules for inheritance, rules for local governance, etc. For 750 years, Norwegians have behaved fairly organized according to ever more modernized versions of this law. This law (and a good portion of luck about the oil found) is part of the reason why Norway is one of the richest countries in the world and one of the most egalitarian. It should rightfully be considered as fundamental for the foundation matrix of Norway. It has shaped how people think, feel and relate, from the level of individuals to families, groups, regions and the state. It has opened some structured ways of communication ("web") where something is allowed and wanted, while else something is forbidden (e.g., incest, violence, thefts, rebellion against the king, etc.).

Is there any content in this communicational web? The web itself is based upon content. It *is* the content. Like: "Disputes between neighbouring peasants should be resolved by …". However, there is a lot of "content" which has not been part of the foundation matrix because it has not been thought of as relevant for public affairs. Also here, we see a historical process. E.g., in most Western democracies there are now rules and regulations for marriage among gay people, something which was unheard about for some decades ago. Content which are not relevant or forbidden or too specialized for the foundation matrix may be thought about and acted upon in the dynamic matrices of families and small groups. In earlier times, family groups were a "free space" for all sorts of behaviour, from sex to domestic violence, dominance and submission. In modern times, e.g., in Norway, much of this behaviour is not allowed any longer. The modern family matrix is not allowed to let violence happen. If so, the child welfare agency interferes. However, there is still a lot of freedom for families to develop their own peculiar matrix, i.e., their typical ways of speaking, acting and relating and this might be more or less conducive for the mental health of the family group members. What might not be openly expressed in the family matrix, may be thought about and shared in other group contexts, like peer groups. Or it might not be expressed at all, being confined to unverbalized parts of the body.

It may also be useful to speak of different foundational webs. In modern societies, the stock exchange is playing an essential role for the economies "to go around". The stock price measures the feelings among investors who have a great impact upon the course of societies. When there is a feeling of optimism (SEEKING), investments and energy go up. When there is a feeling of FEAR for the future, investments and energy go down, in the worst case scenario leading to recession with huge consequences for people. The stock exchange agencies measure these regional and global tendencies thanks to modern IT technology. They rely literally on a digital web that measures feelings. Is this global information web the closest we come to a kind of measurement of (parts of) the global foundation matrix?

The concepts of group mind and matrix in the writings of Foulkes were hardly empirical concepts. They were described in general terms as something that concerned groups in general, and they have hardly been objects for empirical research. Perhaps we should look upon them as concepts that belong more to an early effort at a *philosophy of groups* and that Foulkes was a pioneer in this respect. Such a view makes it all the more relevant trying to reconcile Foulkes's concepts with those of Searle. Searle, in his book *Making the Social World* (2010, p.5), suggests a new philosophy of society

> … namely, the study of the nature of human society itself: what is the mode of existence of social entities such as governments, families, cocktail parties, summer vacations, trade unions, baseball games and passports?

Foulkes would have said that such social entities (mostly groups) come with a matrix. In a general sense it will refer to some structure (communicational web) that unites the group members. Following Searle, we will say that this structure comes as a consequence of the constitutional declaration, i.e., by the deontological powers (rules, norms and regulations) that accompany the declaration. Thereby we reconcile the concepts of matrix, mentalization and the group self. Human groups are constituted by collective intentionality through speech acts that presuppose a mentalizing ability. That is the abstract formula. In practice, when people must relate to each other in certain ways, they become emotionally involved. They develop a relational and communicational network which is specific for the purpose of the group and the particular characters which the group consists of. This network facilitates certain modes of behaviour and suppress other modes (e.g., violent disputes and sexual harassment). By that, the group acquires certain characteristics, similar to personality characteristics. The group matrix may then be likened to the personality matrix, i.e., to the dynamic balance of emotions and attitudes inside each individual which constitutes the self. By that, the concepts of the group matrix and the group self become rather similar. The benefit of the group matrix concept is that it more clearly refers to a *dynamic interplay* between the members of the group. They are in a perpetual emotional interaction. The group self-concept might seem more static. It refers more clearly to the joint purpose of the group. However, we must remind ourselves that the self is not a static thing. It is more profoundly a project of living (with others in groups and societies) composed of conflicting emotional and attitudinal parts, under the umbrella of selfhood and identity. In conclusion we might say that group matrix and group self are related and overlapping concepts. They may be used for different purposes, according to what we would like to emphasize with respect to group dynamics. Foulkes should be appreciated for reminding us that group matrix is something evolutionary ancient. E.g., chimpanzees live in organized groups with a social hierarchy. Obviously, there is a structure there. However, this structure is not mentalized and thus it is static. Chimpanzees are not able to transcend their social structure. They are not able to create a group self that is self-reflective because they lack verbal language, mentalizing abilities and the capacity to create social institutions by speech acts.

Implications and summary

This essay has been mainly conceptual. However, the implications are highly practical. By linking Foulkes' major emphasis on communicational processes in groups to the theories of mentalizing and social ontology, group analytic theory becomes more modern, i.e., more in tune with essential neighbouring disciplines. It opens for a more rational discourse on how to deal with individual and collective mentalizing breakdowns without resorting to outdated metapsychology. Furthermore, it opens for a more flexible approach whereby the conductor might adjust his/her therapeutic style according to the developmental level of the group and its individual and mentalizing challenges. This is especially important for the practice of group analysis outside of private practice, e.g., in the National Mental Health Services.

There are good reasons to contend that group analysis should comprise a broad and flexible approach to group psychotherapy where the conductor adjusts his/her therapeutic style according to the prevailing boundary conditions and level of personality functioning of the participants (Karterud et al., 2024). The question is, what does that mean and require when it comes to clinical realities. In this introductory chapter, I have tried to demonstrate how the theory of mentalizing is the best conceptual tool for understanding the social processes that Foulkes valued the most about group analysis, i.e., the concerted ability to convert psychic symptoms by collective meaningful discourse. In a mentalizing language: To mentalize unmentalized emotions through collective discourse and thereby open for self- and personality development. The series of articles that follow this introduction deal with theoretical and therapeutic challenges of realizing such a collective discourse when the personality problems among the participants are pervasive. By stretching the boundaries for group analysis, we become challenged as to indications for group analysis, its possibilities and limits, its technical components and the grounding concepts related to individual and group ontology (Karterud, 2015). This is a never-ending discussion. This book does not deliver any final conclusions. However, hopefully it might contribute to the development of the field and posit group analysis in a better position for fruitful dialogues with the new conceptualizations of personality disorders as defined by ICD-11. The language of ICD-11's chapter on personality and its disorders is about self and interpersonal functioning:

> Taken together, at the heart of personality functioning (and personality disorder) lies the sense of identity, self-worth, and agency, which can be reciprocally defined by authentic, mutual, and caring relationships throughout life.
>
> (Bach, 2025)

This is the language that will dominate the field for years to come. By being "official" as linked to an internationally agreed upon classificatory system, this "language" will also be the language spoken by health authorities. If we intend to compete over resources, we must be at terms with this language. This language is far from complete. However, it is compatible with the theory I promote in this book. My theory takes it deeper by integrating individual and social ontology and outlining the conditions for healthy individual and collective being. Most importantly, this integration is done with reference to empirical research which will be clarified in the following chapters. Individual and collective mentalizing can be measured, as well as group therapist's interventions. This has far-reaching consequences for training and quality control, which are necessary ingrediencies of any organized activity that claims to benefit the mental health of the population.

In summary, in this essay I have:

- Taken as my departure the incompleteness of group analytic theory in explaining how a collective discourse of a certain kind might help to dissolve symptoms and promote self- and personality development among group members.
- Discussed early versions of psychoanalytic theories of thinking, as found in Freud and Bion, and explained the more modern theory of mentalization which implies a movement from words to narratives.
- By this move, the dependency of the individual upon the collective discourse of his surrounds becomes more apparent.
- The theory I promote substantiates Foulkes claim that "forces" in the group "penetrate the individual to its innermost core" as well as Foulkes' emphasis on communicational processes in therapeutic groups with particular reference to "autistic parts" of the self.
- It clarifies the role of language in making "autistic parts" conscious.
- It clarifies that "forces" in the mind (and group) are manifestations of emotions and their behavioural and social implications.
- It holds that increased consciousness of a certain kind dissolve symptoms and favour personality growth.
- It underlines the role of resonance in the group and the conductor's role in translation.
- It considers language as an evolutionary product of groups which master collective intentionality.
- It asserts that to develop and thrive humans need to be mentalized. And they need to mentalize to thrive in an intersubjective world.
- It reminds us that the social world is not only intersubjective. It is organized by social institutions, e.g., groups of different kinds.
- That these groups are dependent on mentalizing abilities, i.e., the ability to perform and understand certain speech acts that function as constitutive declarations.
- That groups are created by such constitutive declarations which comes with certain rules and obligations ("deontological powers").
- It asserts that due to historical processes (the Zeitgeist), therapeutic groups could be constituted around World War II.
- Thereby it was proved that symptoms could be transformed by a certain collective discourse.
- It claims that the nature of symptoms can be defined as unmentalized emotions and modern theories about their role in the development of personality and self might pave way for a widening scope of group analytic psychotherapy.
- Likewise, the theory of mentalizing in concert with the social ontology definition of groups pave way for a redefinition of the concept of group matrix while cancelling the concept of a group mind.

- The theory holds that group dynamics by necessity is coined by the deontological power (rules and obligations) that comes with constitutive declarations in concert with the interactions due to personal characteristics of the group members (their level of personality functioning and personality style).
- The concepts of the group self and group matrix cover these dynamics.
- Therapeutic groups have potentials for maturation and growth which are displayed by more advanced collective reflective functioning around the purpose of the analytic group which is self- and personality development.
- Being an active and engaged member of such a group has healing implications for the individual member.
- Altogether, these reconceptualizations might open for much needed further developments of group analytic theory and practice.

References

Ainsworth, M., Blehar, M., Waters, E. & Wall, S. (2015). *Patterns of Attachment. A Psychological Study of the Strange Situation*. New York: Psychological Press.

Bach, B. (2025). ICD-11 Personality Disorders. Oxford: Oxford University Press.

Barwick, N. & Weegmann, M. (2018). *Group Therapy. A Group-analytic Approach*. London: Routledge.

Bateman, A., Fonagy, P., Campbell, C., Luyten, P. & Debbanë, M. (2023). *The Cambridge Guide to Mentalization-based Treatment (MBT)*. Cambridge: Cambridge University Press.

Bick, E. (1968/1988). The experience of the skin in early object-relations. In E. Bott Spillius (Ed.), *Melanie Klein Today: Mainly Theory*. London: Routledge.

Bion, W. R. (1961). *Experiences in Groups*. London: Tavistock Publications.

Bion, W. R. (1962). *Learning from Experience*. London: Heineman.

Bion, W. R. (1963). *Elements of Psycho-analysis*. London: Heineman.

Bion, W. R. (1965). *Transformations*. London: Heineman.

Bion, W. R. (1967a). *Second Thoughts. Selected Papers on Psycho-analysis*. New York: Jason Aronson.

Bion, W. R. (1967b). Notes on memory and desire. *The Psychoanalytic Forum*, 2(3).

Bion, W. R. (1975). *A Memoire of the Future. Book One: The Dream*. Rio de Janeiro: Imago Editora Ltd.

Bowlby, J. (1969). *Attachment. Vol. 1, Attachment and Loss*. London: The Hogarth Press.

Bowlby, J. (1973). *Attachment. Vol. 2, Anxiety and Anger*. London: The Hogarth Press.

Bowlby, J. (1980). *Attachment. Vol. 3, Loss: Sadness and Depression*. London: The Hogarth Press.

Burlingame, G. M., McClendon, D. T. & Yang, C. (2018, Dec). Cohesion in group therapy: A meta-analysis. *Psychotherapy (Chic)*, 55(4): 384–398. doi: 10.1037/pst0000173. PMID: 30335452.

Carruthers, P. (2015). *The Centered Mind. What the Science of Working Memory Shows Us About the Nature of Human Thoughts*. Oxford: Oxford University Press.

Cassidy, J. & Shaver, P. R. (1999). *Handbook of Attachment. Theory, Research, and Clinical Application*. New York: The Guildford Press.

Dalal, F. (1998). *Taking the Group Seriously. Towards a Post-Foulkesian Group Analytic Theory*. London: Jessica Kingsley Publisher.
Damasio, A. (2000). *The Feeling of What Happens. Body and Emotions in the Making of Consciousness*. London: Vintage, Random House.
Eagle, M. (2024). *Subjective Experience. Its Fate in Psychology, Psychoanalysis and Philosophy of Mind*. London: Routledge.
Elias, N. (1978). *The Civilizing Process. Vol I: The History of Manners*. Oxford: Blackwell.
Elias, N. (1982). *The Civilizing Process. Vol 2: State Formation and Civilization*. Oxford: Blackwell.
Elias, N. (1996). *The Germans*. Cambridge: Polity Press.
Feinberg, T. E. & Barratt, J. M. (2016). *The Ancient Origins of Consciousness. How the Brain Created Experience*. Cambridge: The MIT Press.
Fonagy, P., Steele, H. & Steele, M. (1991). Maternal representations of attachment during pregnancy predicts the organization of infant-mother attachment at one year of age. *Child Development*, 62(5): 891–905.
Fonagy, P., Target, M., Steele, H. & Steele, M. (1998). Reflective-Functioning Manual Version 5 for Application to Adult Attachment Interviews. https://discovery.ucl.ac.uk/id/eprint/1461016
Fonagy, P., Gergely, G., Jurist, E., et al. (2002). *Affect Regulation, Mentalization and the Development of the Self*. New York: Other Press.
Foulkes, S. H. (1948). *Introduction to Group-Analytic Psychotherapy*. London: Wm. Heinemann Medical Books
Foulkes, S. H. (1964). *Therapeutic Group Analysis*. London: Allen & Unwin.
Foulkes, S. H. & Anthony, E. J. (1957). *Group Psychotherapy: The Psychoanalytic Approach*. Harmondsworth: Penguin Books.
Freud, S. (1895/1966). Project for a scientific psychology. *Standard Edition, vol 1*. London: The Hogarth Press.
Freud, S. (1099). The interpretation of dreams. *The Standard Editions, vol 4-5*. London: The Hogarth Press.
Freud, S. (1913/2004). *Totem and Taboo*. London: Routledge.
Freud, S. (1930). *Civilization and its Discontents. The Standard Edition, vol 21*. London: The Hogarth Press.
Fuchs, T. (2020). The circularity of the embodied mind. *Frontiers in Psychology*, 11: 1707. doi: 10.3389/fpsyg.2020.01707
George, C., Main, M. & Kaplan, N. (1985). *Adult Attachment Interview (AAI) [Database record]*. APA PsycTests. https://doi.org/10.1037/t02879-000
Grice, H. P. (1989). *Studies in the Way of Words*. Boston: Harvard University Press.
Gullestad, S. & Killingmo, B. (2019). *The Theory and Practice of Psychoanalytic Therapy: Listening for the Subtext*. London: Routledge.
Habermas, J. (1984). *The Theory of Communicative Action. Vol 1: Reason and the Rationalization of Society*. Cambridge: Polity Press.
Hegel, G. W. F. (1807/2019). *The Phenomenology of the Spirit*. Cambridge: Cambridge University Press.
Hopper, E. (2014). *The Tripartite Matrix in the Developing Theory and Expanding Practice of Group Analysis. The Social Unconscious in Persons, Groups and Societies: Volume 4*. London: Routledge.

Karterud, S. (1996). The hospital as a therapeutic text. *International Journal of Therapeutic Communities*, 17(2): 125–129.

Karterud, S. (2000). On the scientific foundation of group analysis. *Group Analysis*, 33(4): 514–518.

Karterud, S. (2015a). *Mentalization-Based Group Therapy (MBT-G). A Theoretical, Clinical and Research Manual*. London: Oxford University Press.

Karterud, S. (2015b). On structure and leadership in MBT-G and group analysis. *Group Analysis*, 48(2): 137–149.

Karterud, S. (2023). *Group Analysis. A Modern Synthesis*. London: Routledge.

Karterud, S. & Stone, W. N. (2003). The group self: A neglected aspect of group psychotherapy. *Group Analysis*, 36(1): 7–22.

Karterud, S., Folmo, E. & Kongerslev, M. T. (2019). Personality and the group matrix. *Group Analysis*, 52(4). DOI: 10.1177/0533316418824210

Karterud, S. & Kongerslev, M. T. (2019). A Temperament, Attachment and Mentalization-based (TAM) theory of personality and its disorders. *Frontiers in Psychology*, 10: 518.

Karterud, S. & Kongerslev, M. T. (2021). Psychotherapy of personality disorders needs an integrative theory of personality. *Journal of Psychotherapy Integration*, 31(1): 34–53.

Karterud, S., Gunnarsen, G., Kongerslev, M. T., Staun, L. & Schultz-Venrath, U. (2024). On the relationship between group analysis and mentalization-based group therapy. *Group Analysis*, 58(1). DOI: 10.1177/05333164231218694

Kohut, H. (1971). *The Analysis of the Self.* New York: International Universities Press.

Kohut, H. (1977). *The Restoration of the Self.* New York: International Universities Press.

Main, T. (1946). The hospital as a therapeutic institution. *Bulletin of the Menninger Clinic*, 10: 66–90.

Mitchel, S. (1998). *Relational Concepts in Psychoanalysis. An Integration*. Cambridge: Harvard University Press.

Nitsun, M. (1991). The anti-group: destructive forces in the group and their therapeutic potential. *Group Analysis*, 24(1): 7–30.

Nitsun, M. (1996 [2014]). *The Anti-Group – Destructive Forces in the Group and their Creative Potential*. London: Routledge.

Nitzgen, D. (2024). The cornerstone, once more. In E. Hopper (Ed.), *The Tripartite Matrix in the Developing Theory and Expanding Practice of Group Analysis. The Social Unconscious in Persons, Groups and Societies: Volume 4*. London: Routledge.

Northoff, G. & Panksepp, J. (2008). The trans-species concept of the self and the subcortical-cortical midline system. *Trends in Cognitive Sciences*, 12: 259–264.

Panksepp, J. (1998). *Affective Neuroscience: The Foundations of Humans and Animal Emotions.* Oxford: Oxford University Press.

Panksepp, J. & Biven, L. (2012). *The Archaeology of Mind: Neuroevolutionary Origins of Human Emotions.* New York: W. W. Norton & Company.

Pines, M. (1990). Group analytic psychotherapy and the borderline patient. In B. E., Roth, W. N., Stone, & H. D. Kibel (Eds.), *The Difficult Patient in Group: Group Psychotherapy with Borderline and Narcissistic Disorders* (pp.31–44). Madison: International University Press.

Pines, M. (1996a). Dialogue and selfhood: Discovering connections. *Group Analysis*, 29: 327–341.

Pines, M. (1996b). The self as a group: The group as a self. *Group Analysis*, 29: 183–190.

Pribram, K. H. & Gill, M. M. (1976). *Freud's "Project" Re-assessed.* New York: Basic Books.
Ricoeur, P. (1981). *Hermeneutics and the Human Sciences.* Cambridge: Cambridge University Press.
Ricoeur, P. (1983). *Time and Narrative, vol 1.* Chicago: The University of Chicago Press.
Roberts, B. W., Kuncel, N. R., Shiner, R., Caspi, A. & Goldberg, L. R. (2007). The power of personality: The comparative validity of personality traits, socioeconomic status, and cognitive ability for predicting important life outcomes. *Perspectives on Psychological Science*, 2(4): 313–345.
Schlapobersky, J. (2016). *From the Couch to the Circle: Group-Analytic Psychotherapy in Practice.* London: Routledge.
Schultz-Venrath, U. (2024). *Mentalizing the Body: Integrating Body and Mind in Psychotherapy.* London: Routledge.
Searle, J. R. (2010). *Making the Social World. The Structure of Human Civilization.* Oxford: Oxford University Press.
Stanghellini, G. (2017). *Lost in Dialogue.* Oxford: Oxford University Press.
Stern, D. N. (1985). *The Interpersonal World of the Infant.* New York: Basic Books.
Taylor, C. (1989). *Sources of the Self. The Making of the Modern Identity.* Cambridge: Cambridge University Press.
Taylor, C. (2007). *A Secular Age.* Cambridge: The Belknap Press of Harvard University Press.
Taylor, C. (2016). *The Language Animal.* Cambridge: The Belknap Press of Harvard University Press.
Tomkins, S. S. (1992). *Affect, Imagery, Consciousness. Vol 4: Duplication and Transformation of Information.* New York: Springer.
Tomasello, M. (2014). *A Natural History of Human Thinking.* Cambridge: Harvard University Press.
Tomasello, M. (2019). *Becoming Human: A Theory of Ontogeny.* Cambridge: Belknap Press.
Tronick, E. Z. (2002). *Emotions and Emotional Communication in Infants.* London: Routledge
Whitaker, D. S. (1981). A nuclear conflict and group focal conflict model for integrating individual and group-level phenomena in psychotherapy groups. In M. Pines & L. Rafaelsen (Eds.), *The Individual and the Group: Boundaries and Interrelations in Theory and Practice.* New York: Plenum Press.

Chapter 2

The group self

A neglected aspect of group psychotherapy

Sigmund Karterud and Walter Stone

Abstract

The authors explore and expand on Heinz Kohut's concept "the group self", which is related to, yet different from the concepts "intersubjective field" and "group matrix". The group self is defined as a collective project with inherent ambitions, ideals and resources. From this perspective, the authors discuss group-as-a-whole phenomena, empathy, aspects of group development and the kind of discourse which is appropriate for group psychotherapy. This particular discourse should contain multiple selfobject functions as well as aspects of otherness not accounted for by the selfobject concept. Partaking in this discourse have a beneficial effect by itself which justifies a concept of "discursive selfobject function". This selfobject function is of a partial supra-individual nature. Two clinical vignettes illustrate aspects of group self development and fear of depletion of the group self.

In the last two decades self psychology has exerted considerable influence on group psychotherapy, particularly when applied to understanding clinical phenomena and therapeutic technique. However, to a large extent this has been an application of dyadic self psychology theory and principles to the group situation. In this paper we will discuss a more radical position by addressing the concept of the group as a whole from a self psychological perspective. As we shall see, this turn will illuminate some dim aspects of groups, but also reveal some shortcomings in self psychological theory itself.

The group self

Kohut was not particularly favourable to group psychotherapy (Arensberg, 1998), but he was preoccupied with historical group processes. In the essay Creativeness, Charisma, Group Psychology: Reflections on the Self-Analysis of Freud (Kohut, 1976), he introduced the concept of "the group self". He suggested that "we posit the existence of a certain psychological configuration with regard to the group – let us call it the 'group self' – which is analogous to the self of the individual" (pp. 420–421). In the accompanying footnote, Kohut writes, "The psychoanalytic

DOI: 10.4324/9781003625810-2

concept of the self, however – whether it refers to the self of an individual or to the self of a person as a member of a group or, as a 'group self' to the self of a stable association of people – concerns a structure which dips into the deepest reach of the psyche" (p. 420). He adds, "The basic patterns of a nuclear group self (the group's central ambitions and ideals) account not only for the continuity and the cohesion of the group but also determines its most important actions" (p. 420). Kohut did not develop these ideas theoretically any further although some of his essays, in particular "On Leadership" (Kohut, 1985), contain the group self as an implicit presupposition. Theoretically speaking, the group self is thus an underdeveloped concept. In this paper we will try to give clinical meaning to the concept.

The group-as-a-whole – as object, agent, selfobject and self

In the group psychotherapy literature, the common use of the term "group-as-a-whole" is ambiguous. Firstly, it refers to the group-as-a-whole conceived as an *object*. This usage refers to group members experiential reports and behaviour which suggest that they experience the group as an entity which resembles so-called internal objects. This usage dates back to Bion (1959) who claimed that the ultimate reason for basic assumption phenomena, was the group's resemblance (in the mind of the members) with primitive internal objects. According to this tradition one speaks of the group as an idealised ("good") mother/breast or alternatively as a persecutory or devouring ("bad") mother/breast (Durkin, 1964; Scheidlinger, 1974).

Secondly, one has referred to the group-as-a-whole *as agent* (or subject). This usage is displayed in group-as-a-whole interpretations, such as "the group tends to avoid...", "the problem for the group is...", "the group tends to rid itself of painful conflicts by...", etc. This second usage is closer to a notion of an (agential) group self. However, group psychotherapists have (rightly) maintained an ambivalent attitude towards the group as agent. Group-agential interpretations are probably used rather frequently, yet the theoretical grounds for such interpretations are not satisfactory within existing paradigms since accepting the group as agent is close to investing the group with a supra-individual mind.

Thirdly, the group-as-a-whole has been conceived of as a selfobject (Stone, 1992). This refers to experiences of being strengthened by group membership in itself. Nowadays many will refer to attachment needs in order to explain this phenomenon. Later in this paper we will relate the group-as-selfobject to the supra-individual nature of group discourse.

Fourth, the group-as-a-whole can be approached from the perspective of the self, as will be outlined in the following paragraphs.

The group-as-a-whole conceived as object, agent/subject, selfobject or self refers to different aspects of experience and behaviour in groups. These concepts are more experience near than the concepts of group matrix and interpersonal field. The group matrix refers to the conscious and unconscious communicational network in the group (Foulkes & Anthony, 1957; Foulkes, 1973). It is related to established group norms and group solutions (Whitaker & Lieberman, 1964). Thus, the group matrix is impregnated with an interpersonal "direction" so to speak. An intersubjective field is more abstract. It lacks a foundation in an interpersonal project, which we will elaborate in the next paragraph. It is crucial to underline that neither the concept of matrix nor the intersubjective field catches the agential aspect of the group-as-a-whole. *It does not make sense to attribute intentions to a matrix or to an intersubjective field.* How can we properly say that a group *wants something*, without violate ordinary language rules? In our opinion, claiming that there exist needs on a group-as-a-whole level, presupposes a concept of a group self.

The group self as project

Whatever are the reasons for people being together, they will necessarily construct meanings and purposes for their togetherness. This quality, the purpose of togetherness, is fundamental to group formation, and, we will add, a fundamental quality of the group self. With reference to Sartre's (1943) notion of a fundamental project for the individual existence/self, we will argue that this sense of purpose of being together is part of a larger phenomenon, of a *collective project.* People come together in order to achieve something, and the group self is the conscious and unconscious structure that embodies the project. The project contains both the rational deliberative part of group formation ("I join this group because of my interest in the subject matter") and a host of unconscious motivations (e.g., attachment needs).

The supra-individual qualities of groups are consequences of the collective nature of the project. Groups do not contain any supra-individual group mind, but a supra-individual project. The project consists of certain ambitions, ideals and resources embedded in a specific history (similar to the individual self), and the project can be carried out on all levels of sophistication. Thus, one is justified to speak of a restricted and primitive versus a mature group self and a disorganised versus an organised group self. The group self is typically composed of a core member subgroup that, more than other members, profoundly identifies with the ambitions and ideals of the project (Kohut, 1985). They are the main spokespersons for the group qua project. They act on behalf of the group self. Experientially they can have difficulties in differentiating between their personal self and their part of the group self. The group project can become identical to the personal life project. An insult to the group will then be perceived as an insult to the personal self.

The concept of project resolves the problem of the agential aspect of groups. As a collective supra-individual project, we are justified to say that the group needs and wants something and resists other things. *What* it wants and resists depends on the nature of the project and the group's interactions with the surroundings. As with the individual self, a group self is full of shortcomings and conflicts and contains an unconscious domain as well as a conscious rational part. These conscious and unconscious conflicts and shortcomings *in the perspective of the needs and the aims of the group self*, in our opinion, justify group-as-a-whole interpretations.

It follows from taking the needs and the aims of the group self seriously, that the question of the future appears as a legitimate theme also at the level of the group-as-a-whole. Aspirations and fears of the future are powerful motivational forces for group actions. Without a perspective of the future, things become meaningless. Where should the concern for the future of the group be located, if not in the group self?

The nature of the project defines the *kind of discourse* that is most appropriate for the group. There are quite different discourses (defined as communicational patterns, attitudes, belief systems, etc.) in a Hells Angels group compared to a scientific committee. The discourse concept covers much of the same terrain as matrix and intersubjective field but takes it a bit further. The discourse also conveys a supra-individual structure. It is akin to Wittgenstein's notion of *language games*. The language game of contemporary psychotherapy is quite different from the language game of bridge. The crucial point is that the established discourse, or language game, which tradition has established within a profession, will set the stage for the events to be displayed. One is not personal author of an established discourse tradition, e.g., psychodynamic group psychotherapy. One is an actor within the rules set by the discourse, and in a certain respect one can say that one is played with by the discourse (group). In our opinion, this points to a limitation in contemporary intersubjective theory, where the intersubjective field is conceived as created by the protagonist's ways of organising experience according to different cognitive-affective schemata (Stolorow, Brandchaft, & Atwood, 1987). This definition does not give sufficient space for the supra-individual forces embedded in the operative discourse tradition.

The project of (long term) psychodynamic group psychotherapy is promoting self understanding and self development for the members. The main task of the group therapist is to recruit members to understand and identify with the kind of discourse rules and paradigms of understanding that are most appropriate for this project. By basic discourse rules we mean typically group psychotherapy rules such as regular attendance, commitment, no outside contact, free and open communication, etc. (Rutan & Stone, 2000). By discourse paradigms of understanding we mean a paradigmatic way of attributing meaning to the current group events. Adherents to different schools of group psychotherapy may share basic discourse rules but differ in paradigms of understanding.

In our opinion, it is crucial for *the discourse of self-understanding and self-development*, to pay due attention to the themes which are explicated in the self psychology tradition, such as the basic needs of the self, empathy, the significance of selfobject functions, the repetitive and selfobject transferences, empathic and selfobject failures, etc. During treatment members gradually learn aspects of the language of self-understanding. In particular they will learn to appreciate selfobject functions from other members (and the therapist) and to identify and manage their own experiences of selfobject failures.

However, in addition to selfobject functions that members (or the therapist) perform for each other, we would like to emphasise a kind of selfobject function which have been unrecognised, and which cannot be attributed to acts of care and understanding from one person to another. We will label this selfobject function as a *discoursive selfobject function.* We contend that when people feel strengthened after a group session, this is partly due to participating in a kind of discourse, rich in cognitive and affective perspectives and nuances, that the individual is unable to perform for himself. This conversation, which enables the individual to understand more fully intrapsychic, interpersonal and group events, is not attributable to specific individuals. It is a *supra-individual discourse event.*

In the following we will comment upon the topics of empathy and developmental stages involved in the establishment of a discourse of self-understanding and self-development and thereafter discuss two clinical vignettes.

Aspects of group development

Most contemporary group psychotherapists adhere to a progressive theory of group development, i.e. a development from a state of low coherence and immaturity to a state of maturity and coherence. A progressive view is analogous to the development of the individual self (from an emergent sense of self to a consolidated and competent self) as well as the development of whole nations (from despotism, slavery and injustice to liberalism and democracy). We shall not discuss the details of developmental subphases but restrict ourselves to issues of paramount importance for the formation of a group self.

What developments and interactions are necessary for members to feel that belonging to the group will be emotionally satisfying, will help them feel that they belong to a worthwhile enterprise, that they will feel more powerful, more complete, more able to pursue their personal goals and stand-up for their ideals? In the opening phase of group formation, members are concerned about how to proceed and how the experience can feel safe and trustworthy. Myers (1996) asserts that members' initial anxiety is that others will fail to provide mirroring. Joining a group evokes feelings of relative helplessness and narcissistic imbalance. According to Myers this is countered by mobilising an idealising transference to the therapist, and by extension to the group as a whole. Members attempt to orient themselves by obtaining information from the leader on how to make the experience useful, which they hope will not only reduce anxiety but provide direction. Inevitably these efforts will be frustrated and fail, resulting in experiences of anxiety and disequilibrium (Stone, 1985, 1995).

In our opinion the term "idealisation" is too ambiguous to capture the essence of the *orientation phase* dynamics. What is labelled idealisation covers an existential terrain that extends from submission to idealisation proper. We contend that submission is the predominant mode in the orientation phase. It represents defensive self-structures which are activated due to the fear of retraumatization. Idealising selfobject transferences usually occur much later. They develop slowly after the resolution of the conflict ("storming") phase (Karterud, 1999).

We believe that differentiating between submission and idealising selfobject transferences is crucial and points to a problem in contemporary self psychology. It is no longer in vogue to talk about defensive self-structures. In contemporary self psychology, one has moved from optimal frustration (Kohut & Seitz, 1963) to other ways of conceptualising "optimal" therapist-patient exchange, e.g., optimal responsiveness, optimal provision, optimal restraint and facilitating responsiveness (Bacal, 1985; Siegel, 1999).

Although we sympathise with these efforts, we worry that these conceptualisations blur the ingredient of frustration which is inherent in analytic relations. The phenomenon of submission pinpoints these different attitudes: Should one frustrate or provide gratification for submissive needs? In group psychotherapy a considerable element of frustration is inevitable. However, group therapists differ in their technique and the way they theorise about it. In our opinion, self-understanding and self-development requires an oscillation between deconstruction of defensive self-structures and construction of authentic self-structures by reactivation and working through of archaic selfobject transferences.

Initially, the group is (rightly) perceived as therapist centred. The clinician's main task is to guide members through a phase of partial resolution of individual and collective submissiveness, to mobilise anger towards old and new authoritative figures, to activate the striving for autonomy, to facilitate a fresh series of negotiations of the basic rules and grounding discourse rules, whereby the members can properly say they "own" the group, which means that the group self is grounded in a collective project.

Since the therapist's attitude is deliberately group-oriented and interpretative, and not fundamentally individualistic-supportive, he/she will inevitably evoke experiences of selfobject failures (i.e., narcissistic injuries). Members' responses may be withdrawal or exploring connections with emotionally available others, i.e. those who can recognise and appreciate what the person emotionally needs. However, withdrawal from the therapist is seldom complete, and patients' experiences of the therapist as predictable, dependable and reliable while listening, attempting to understand and respond, provides a backdrop to which patients can return when peer relations are aversive.

It is each person's inner experience to the response of the therapist and members that lead to stabilising or enhancing the self. Under optimal circumstances trust develops and increased risk-taking follows. These interactions create group norms and the slow development of a discourse that promotes self-understanding and self-development (Stone, 1996).

The therapist's abdication from gratifying submissive needs "forces" patients to address their fellow group members. By turning to others, individuals have a fair chance to find repositories for a wide variety of human needs, be they "defensive", "perverse" or "sympathetic". The result is covert and overt subgroups and alliances, and we are in agreement with Agazarian (1997) who emphasises that a substantial part of the dynamics is played out (at least in the earlier phases of group development) between subgroups. Subgrouping is an important source of stabilising a threatened self in group psychotherapy.

This leads us to some remarks on *the significance of the other* in group psychotherapy. Self psychology has traditionally emphasised the selfobject function of the other. We fully agree with the view that selfobject availability is the single most important ingredient in a psychotherapeutic group culture. If patients do not modify defences and permit experiences of being respected, listened to, cared for, confirmed, understood in depth, supported, finding crucial similarities in others, finding crucial aspects to idealise, etc., – group psychotherapy will not work. To use Kohut's phrase, there would be insufficient oxygen for the group to develop or even survive. However, *selfobject experiences are necessary but not sufficient prerequisites for growth.* The others are needed for several other purposes, of which we will emphasise two. 1) The others are needed as repositories for projections. Without the other(s) there would be no possibility for enactments of the dramas of the inner world. Group psychotherapy presupposes a willingness to take on projected roles and become actors in externalised dramas. When individual members hate, despise and envy each other, they usually do not realise that they also need others in such roles. The individual will co-construct with others a wide range of transferential scenarios (Gans & Alonso, 1998). 2) The others are needed as sheer otherness. A group consisting of mere selfobjects (which can hardly be conceived) would be extremely dull and boring. The others are needed to bring in diversities and differences, other and opposing point of views, other perspectives on the world. Without this otherness, no deconstruction could be possible.

These elements are somewhat neglected in contemporary self psychological theory. The concept of "adversarial selfobjects" tries to repair this theoretical lacuna (Wolf, 1988). However, this concept is a contradiction in terms. In our opinion, selfobjects can never be "adversarial". In Kohut's theory, selfobject experiences are univocally positive experiences (conscious and unconscious) that strengthens the self. The crucial point is that the self needs more than selfobject experiences. It also needs resistance, opposition and disagreement. It even needs selfobject failures. It is only through a dialogue with another self that the self can come to know itself and develop (Karterud, 1998).

The developmental aim of psychodynamic group psychotherapy is thus to establish a group culture which has a rich potential for selfobject experiences, which contains the courage to set in motion inner dramas in the here and now, and a tolerance for diversities and differences. This represents an ideal group self, and this ideal group self should be considered as a *regulatory idea*. It is seldom fully realised, but the striving for it is worthwhile since the striving to establish an ideal group self is the very activity through which the individual self comes to a fuller understanding of itself and proceeds with development. A group that has lost the "memoirs of the ideal group self", has lost crucial perspectives of the future. It will be locked in depression or chronic internal fighting which will lead nowhere.

Empathy

We fully agree with Kohut that empathy is the primary mode of access to the inner world of the patients (as well as the group as a whole). Empathy is the effort to understand the other "from within". The ability to engage in a sustained immersion with the other's perspective on the world is a prerequisite for psychotherapeutic work. The challenges for the group psychotherapist in this respect are enormous. One is presumed to be in empathic contact with 6–8 persons, the ongoing interactions as well as the state of the group self at each moment of time. It goes without saying that this is an impossible task. Consequently, the therapist's empathic failures are inevitable, making his/her ability to detect and address these failures all the more important (Stone, 2001).

However, what we would like to emphasise here is the relation between empathy and theory. Schematically, the very operation of empathy involves an emotional attunement as well as a cognitive element of constructing meaning to the perceptions of the other. The cognitive element is necessarily suffused by "preunderstanding" (Gadamer, 1960). One cannot understand another without presuppositions, and group therapists' presuppositions are replete with theoretical constructs. Since, theoretically, group events are systemic events, the cognitive elements of the empathy operations come to the forefront. One cannot understand a systemic event without a preunderstanding of the structure and dynamics of the system.

Contemporary group psychotherapists explore a group event from at least three perspectives: From the perspective of the individual intrapsychic, from interpersonal transactions, and from the group-as-a-whole; all three perspectives contain hypotheses about the unconscious operations at work. This complex perspectivity is a hallmark of modernity. It was not accessible to previous generations simply because it was unthought of. When contemporary group psychotherapists "spontaneously" oscillate between these perspectives in their effort to understand, and by these "manoeuvres" understand more fully, this does not imply that, as individuals, they are more empathetic than say Hippocrates or Joseph Pratt, but that these theoretically listening perspectives are internalised through tradition and training. They have become a part of his/hers "natural" presuppositions. By this we mean to underline that theoretical presuppositions are intrinsically embedded in the very operation of empathy.

The most difficult empathic operation, in our opinion, is empathy with the group self. This is so because the therapist is such an integral part of the group self. Initially the group self is solely a "phantasy" in his own mind. He contains the ambitions to carry out a project which he labels psychodynamic group psychotherapy. When he materialises this phantasy to a concrete group, he will realise that the externalisation of his internal project will take on unexpected forms and courses.

He will be caught in a drama much larger than he could ever have conceived. The two main "debates", or negotiation processes, that inevitably will evolve is: 1) The debate between the members about the why, how and where of the group, and 2) the debate between the members and the therapist on the same issues. The guiding principles for the therapist in these negotiation processes are (often vague and contradictory) ideas about the ideal group self. He wants to implement various aspects of the kind of discourse which we have discussed above. However, he will eventually realise that the group self that emerges through the negotiations in the group often will deviate considerably from his own ideals. The larger group self thus contains a tension between the ideals and aspirations of the therapist (as well as those of the members) and the actual discourse that is established as a result of a large series of "negotiations". When this gap is considerable, the therapist may lose empathic contact with several elements in these dialectics. He may "forget" several of his initial ambitions and ideals and resort to supportive strategies; he may resign, "these patients are too disturbed"; he may act out his impatience and disappointment, etc. In our opinion, it is crucial for group vitality that the therapist endures the pain and the grief located in the space between the ideals and the factual discourse, and keep an empathic contact with both aspects, using this tension as a productive ground for thought.

Clinical illustrations

Example 1: Members of a six-person outpatient group struggled to enter into a meaningful dialogue. The meetings were often characterised by extended periods of silence. Two members were almost totally silent. Consistent efforts focused on understanding the meaning of this rather sterile group formation were not productive.

Eunice, a single woman, with a diagnosis of borderline personality disorder, was the most vocal member. She complained about almost all aspects of the treatment: the starkness of the consulting room, the lack of recognition of her special sensitivities and assets, and the silences and stilted interaction in the sessions (in many respects the sessions reflected her marked social isolation and complaints that those in her work environment did not appreciate her talents or abilities). She spoke of both the great relief she felt when she left the city for a business meeting, and yet she said that she wanted the group to succeed because she needed a group to make her life meaningful.

Depicting her perception of the therapist's responsibility, Eunice reported a dream in which the therapist was shutting off the group's view of the outside world by pulling the blinds over a picture window. The members' associations contrasted the relatively free chatter in the period before the start of the session to their silence when the therapist entered the room. They attributed their behaviour to his disapproval of their "social" discussion. This dream helped the therapist appreciate the personal limitations of the members.

In supervision, the therapist began to appreciate that the members appeared to need an extensive period of "social" discussion. They were not yet prepared to take the step of a psychodynamic group in exploring within group interactions the meaning of their discourse. The group self they hoped for (which was compatible with their level of self-development) seemed at odds with that of their therapist. With this understanding, the clinician was able to interact with the members at the level they functioned. This "loosened" the discourse, which, over an extended period, led to their nascent capacity to self-reflect and examine their relationships.

Comment: This example illustrates a countertransference that arose specifically from the clinician's notion of an ideal group self formation. He overestimated members' capacities and became impatient. Eunice's dream brought to the surface the rift between patients and therapist regarding an ideal group self.

Example 2: A long-term outpatient group, led by one of the authors, composed of four men and three women, was focused on two somewhat overlapping issues. The primary focus was on Eve, a senior member, who had shown substantial growth and had been wondering about ending treatment. The group reacted to her plan to terminate with pleasure, recognising her achievement as she evolved from a person who barely spoke to one who would take a leadership role. Several members expressed envy of her achievements. Ken expressed regret and wished that she would not leave.

In the context of Eve's processing her plan to terminate, several events impinged upon the group boundary or alluded to disrupted relationship: A patient who had precipitously terminated the group several years previously began a brief affair with a current member, and Aaron who had planned to end his loveless marriage, announced he could not deliver divorce papers and felt stuck. The members listened to descriptions of these events, which the therapist linked to Eve's departure, but they seemed unable to reflect upon their inner experience. The therapist became aware of a sense of doom – the group would not function with Eve's departure.

Near the end of the session prior to Eve's departure, as Aaron described his wife's incompetence in purchasing a new car, the discussion became highly critical of used car dealers. These were unscrupulous individuals who manipulated, lied, withheld information and took people in. Aaron acknowledged that his wife had nearly made a very bad deal, as a symptom of her behaviour. In the final minutes of the session, tension erupted as several members encouraged Aaron to patch up the marriage while others suggested he move towards divorce.

The therapist felt that he had been unable to fit this discussion into any coherent framework. Rather, he found himself unable to concentrate on the process and was preoccupied with what the group would be like after Eve departed. Only in retrospect, did he realise that the countertransference arose from his anticipation that the group self would be disrupted, and instead of a lively and interactive group he was anticipating an emotionally unengaging, concrete discourse.

Comment: The session illustrates what we believe to be the impact of the unconscious phantasy that the group discourse was about to be shattered. Segalla (1996) asserts "the need to associate/affiliate with a group cannot be satisfied without some *capacity to experience the self as equal to the requirements of members*" (italics in original) (p. 264). In the therapist's mind, Eve's leadership had obscured others' capacities. The therapist feared the members could not maintain a psychodynamic group self. His ability to empathise with the members and with the disruption to the group was temporarily impaired.

These vignettes bring into focus the two threads we have been addressing in this paper: that of the theory of the group self and the role of theory in our use of empathy. The first example illustrates the precarious process of integrating (a subgroup of) silent individuals in a developing group self, while simultaneously fearing that "the owner of the group", the therapist, would resist the elements of autonomous action ("social talk") contained therein. This group is on the way from a dependent group self to a more autonomous group self. The second example concerns an upcoming loss and fear of depletion of the group self and focuses on the therapist's phantasies and resultant countertransference response.

Conclusions

1. Group psychotherapy is in a privileged position to explore and expand on Kohut's concept "the group self", which has been ignored by contemporary self psychology.
2. The group self is conceptually related to, but different from "intersubjective field" and "group matrix".
3. The group self is defined as a collective project and justifies the agential perspective that is implicit in group-as-a-whole interpretations.
4. Exploration of the concept leads to a selfobjectfunction which has not previously been acknowledged – "a discoursive selfobjectfunction".
5. Contemporary self psychology has neglected the significance of "the other" outside the realm of selfobjectfunctions. An examination of the "discourse of self-understanding and self-development" reveals the significance of the other(s) as 1) repository of projections, and 2) otherness as a necessary ingredient in a true dialogue.
6. The very operation of empathy is suffused by theoretical presuppositions.
7. Empathy with the group self is particularly difficult since it implies a reflective empathy with the discrepancies between the therapist's ambitions and ideals and that of the factual group discourse.
8. The clinical vignettes highlight difficulties with the development of an autonomous group self and the impending loss of a vital part of a group self and the members' and the therapist's responses to threats of fragmentation.

References

Agazarian, Y. M. (1997). *Systems-Centred Therapy for Groups*. New York: Guilford Press

Arensberg, F. (1998). A consideration of Kohut's views on group psychotherapy. In I. N. H. Harwood & M. Pines (Eds.), *Self Experiences in Group: Intersubjective and Self Psychological Pathways to Human Understanding*. London: Jessica Kingsley.

Bacal, H. A. (1985). Optimal responsiveness and the therapeutic process. In A. Goldberg (Ed.), *Progress in Self Psychology, (vol 1)*. Hillsdale: The Analytic Press.

Bion, W. R. (1959). *Experiences in Groups*. New York: Basic Books.

Durkin, H. (1964). *The Group in Depth*. New York: International Universities Press.

Foulkes, S. H. (1973). The group as matrix of the individual's mental life. In L. R. Wolberg & E. K. Schwartz (Eds.), *Group Therapy 1973*. New York: Intercontinental Medical Book Corporation.

Foulkes, S. H. & Anthony, E. J. (1957). *Group Psychotherapy: The Psychoanalytical Approach*. Harmondsworth: Penguin Books.

Gadamer, H. G. (1960). *Truth and Method*. London: Sheed & Ward (1989).

Gans, J. S. & Alonso, A. (1998). Difficult patients: Their construction in group therapy. *International Journal of Group Psychotherapy*, 48, 311–326.

Karterud, S. (1998). The group self, empathy, intersubjectivity and hermeneutics: A group analytic perspective. In I. N. H. Harwood & M. Pines (Eds.), *Self Experiences in Group: Intersubjective and Self Psychological Pathways to Human Understanding*. London: Jessica Kingsley.

Karterud, S. (1999). *Gruppeanalyse og psykodynamisk gruppepsykoterapi*. Oslo: Pax forlag.

Kohut, H. (1976). Creativeness, charisma, group psychology. In J. E. Gedo & G. H. Pollock (Eds.), *Freud: The Fusion of Science and Humanism*. New York: International Universities Press.

Kohut, H. (1985). *Self Psychology and the Humanities*. New York: W.W. Norton & Company.

Kohut, H. & Seitz, P. F. D. (1963). Concepts and theories of psychoanalysis. In P. H. Ornstein (Ed.), *The Search for the Self, vol 1*. New York: International Universities Press (1978).

Myers, S. M. (1996). Group therapy and disorders of the self. *Group Analysis*, 29: 219–227.

Rutan, J. S. & Stone, W. N. (2000). *Psychodynamic Group Psychotherapy*, (3rd edition). New York: Guilford.

Sartre, J. P. (1943). *Being and Nothingness*. New York: Washington Square Press (1966).

Scheidlinger, S. (1974). On the concept of the mother-group. *International Journal of Group Psychotherapy*, 24: 417–428.

Segalla, R. A. (1996). The unbearable embeddedness of being: Self psychology, intersubjectivity and large group experiences. *Group*, 20: 257–271.

Siegel, A. M. (1999). The optimal conversation: A concern about current trends within self psychology. In A. Goldberg (Ed.), *Pluralism in Self Psychology. Progress in Self Psychology, vol 15*. Hillsdale: The Analytic Press.

Stolorow, R. D., Brandchaft, B. & Atwood, G. (1987). *Psychoanalytic Treatment: An Intersubjective Approach*. Hillsdale: Analytic Press.

Stone, W. N. (1985). The curative fantasy in group psychotherapy. *Group*, 9: 3–14.

Stone, W. N. (1992). The clinical application of self psychology theory. In R. H. Klein, H. S. Bernard, & D. L. Singer (Eds.), *Handbook of Contemporary Group Psychotherapy*. Madison: International Universities Press.

Stone, W. N. (1995) Frustration, anger and the significance of alter-ego transferences in group psychotherapy. *International Journal of Group Psychotherapy*, 45: 287–302.

Stone, W. N. (1996). Self psychology and the higher mental functioning hypothesis: Complementary theories. *Group Analysis*, 29: 169–181.

Stone, W. N. (2001). The role of the therapist's affect in the detection of empathic failures, misunderstandings and injury. *Group*, 25: 3–14.

Whitaker, D. S. & Lieberman, M. A. (1964). *Psychotherapy through the Group Process*. New York: Atherton.

Wolf, E. S. (1988). *Treating the Self: Elements of Clinical Self Psychology*. New York: Guilford.

Chapter 3

Dreams as portraits of self and group interaction

Walter N. Stone and Sigmund Karterud

Abstract

Dreams presented in group psychotherapy portray different aspects of the dialectic between the group and the individual. A self psychological perspective emphasises the interplay between the current self-state of the group as a whole and the selfobject needs of the individual. With this focus in mind, the therapist should help the group to deepen the awareness and capacity to reflect on emerging new abilities ("forward edge"). Dream imagery and the needed human responsiveness can actualise these abilities and thus help the individual and the group to break and transform chains of repetition compulsion. The approach is illustrated with two clinical examples. The article is the first to bridge concepts and ideation from the self psychology tradition with that of mentalizing. In the reflections on dreams and group discourse the authors refer to psychic equivalence and pretend mode. They use pretend mode in a positive sense, as that kind of imagining and thinking which is linked to play and which signals a bridge towards more mature representational thinking. There is also a reference to Winnicott's notion of "playing with reality". The ability to play with words (and feelings) is crucial for a mature analytic group. A deadly serious group is (still) bound to psychic equivalence thinking which overestimates the significance of subjective experiences. The acceptance of contrasting perspectives moves the group and the persons therein to an exploration of the interface of fantasy and reality, the inner and the outer world. It is a quality of group communication and discourse that favours individual and collective developments.

From the time of Freud's (1900/1953) classical monograph, dreams have been regarded as avenues into the unconscious world of wishes, conflicts and defences. The interpretative task, with the aid of the patient's associations, was traditionally to decode unconscious elements that the dream disguised. In contrast, self psychology has focused its attention on the dream's representation of the self, and self in relation to others, others in the past and in the present. As Ornstein (1987) wrote, "The dream is always about the self; that is, the dream always presents various aspects of self-experience to the dreamer's attention" (p. 101).

DOI: 10.4324/9781003625810-3

Atwood and Stolorow (1984) highlight the value of conceptualizing dreams as concrete symbols that "serve to actualize a *particular* [sic] organization of experience in which specific configurations of self and object ... are dramatized and affirmed" (p. 103). These authors suggest that "dream symbols bring the state of the self into focal awareness, with a feeling of conviction and reality that can only accompany sensory perceptions" (pp. 104–105). Further emphasising the integrative and synthetic function of dream imagery for the self, Fosshage (1997) posits that "the superordinate function of dreams is the development, maintenance (regulation), and when necessary, restoration of psychic process ... and [psychological] organization" (p. 433). He emphasises that affect regulation in sustaining or restoring a disrupted self is a primary function of dreams.

In individual psychoanalytic psychotherapy dreams are progressively coloured by the transference involvement as the therapeutic process deepens. In group psychotherapy dreams become responses to the highly complex social situation of the group, of which the dreamer is a part. The clinical literature has added the concept of group dreams, which it defines as dreams containing concrete or "slightly" disguised references in the manifest content to the group (Karterud, 1992). We suggest that most dreams reported in psychotherapy groups portray different aspects of the dialectic interplay between the group and the individual self.

Group dreams from self psychological perspectives

Dreams, viewed from the lens of self psychology, may express exhibitionistic/grandiose strivings or searching for selfobject affirmation (Stone & Whitman, 1977) or wishes for merger with an idealised selfobject (Stone, 1992). Dreams reported in the group may reflect a wish for a response from particular members or as a representation of the dreamer's inner experience of the group-as-a-whole (Harwood, 1998). Group dreams may also reflect resistances to engaging in the group which, in turn, may represent earlier family or group experiences that were traumatic or failed to provide necessary optimal responsiveness (Bacal, 1985). Group dreams can also portray the dissolution or disintegration of the group as manifested by objects breaking apart and which may be stimulated by actual or anticipated loss (a member terminating or an interruption of regular sessions) or by reawakening of earlier losses such as death or divorce.

Threats to the self may arise from numerous sources in the group. Violations of group norms or boundaries, such as an extra-group liaison or chronic tardiness, may be experienced consciously or subliminally and be reflected symbolically in the dream as broken fences or crumbling walls. Affect overstimulation, as in intense erotic attractions, primitive envy, or idealization, can fuel dream imagery of floods or tornadoes. At a less dramatic level, narcissistic injury arising from seemingly innocuous interactions, such as being offered advice or asking a question that has just been answered, can impact on the member's inner image of the group. Discourse of this nature, characteristic of early stages of group development, is often accompanied by the recipient's experience of unverbalised shame, which may shatter his/her trust in the group. A dream may be the patient's communication of this kind of disruptive experience.

We have previously suggested that there are three relevant perspectives to group-as-a-whole phenomena that may be reflected in dreams: (1) the group as object such as "bad mother" symbolised, for example, as a dangerous or unavailable individual or as an empty building; (2) the group as selfobject that provides supportive functions for the self, reflected, for example, by a family eating a sumptuous meal; and (3) the group self. These perspectives are not mutually exclusive (Karterud, 1998). To the contrary, they enrich each other, as we will try to demonstrate in our clinical examples.

The group self perspective, initially described by Kohut (1976), refers to the collective, supra-individual project on which all members, at least partially, have agreed to collaborate. As part of self, individuals internalise the values, aims, hopes, ideals, and goals of their groups. The project of psychotherapy groups is to enhance self-understanding and self-development through intimate involvement with a limited number of peers and a therapist. The group self carries the ideals of free and open communication, trust in the dialogue, mutual respect and concern, a sense of fairness, and being part of a supportive community (Karterud & Stone, 2003). We believe these ideals are grounded in an evolutionary concern for the self as an interwoven part of groups. These ideals, however, are continuously being undermined by withdrawal, suspiciousness, hostility, greed, envy, rivalry, hate, and craving for revenge. Trying to resolve these tensions on an individual as well as a group self level constitutes a central theme in the therapeutic process.

Thus, as described above, injuries to the self could also be understood as damage to the group self. The termination of a valued group member, for example, likely would carry meaning at multiple levels, including loss at the level of the group and therefore a depletion of the group self resulting from a sense of loss of the departing person's contributions to the group's work. Exploration of self-depletion or fragmentation dreams would be incomplete without considering the possibilities of their also representing a shift in the state of the group self.

Therapeutic considerations

From the perspective of a self-psychologically informed clinician, the purpose of addressing dreams is to help members gain understanding in the fluctuations of their self states, their need for human responsiveness, and emergent possibilities of new ways of being. This would include self-protective, self-restorative, and self-enhancing processes.

Livingston (2001) suggests that dreams presented in groups can never be fully analysed in the classical sense. "The value of working with dreams in group is not the opportunity for completeness and an orderly working through. The value that we can see clearly is in the aliveness and deepening of group process" (p. 24). In addition to representations of the individual's self or group self stage, dreams may metaphorically depict aspects of the treatment process. Sequences may portray aspects of member's self or perceptions of the group interactions as successive scenes.

The self psychological model of pathology is that of developmental arrest, not of inner conflict (Kohut, 1984). Patients not only repeat their developmental difficulties in order to master old conflicts, but they also attempt developmental thrusts. Tolpin (2002) has labelled these "presentations" as "trailing" and "forward" edge. She depicts the tentative nature of the forward edge with the expression "tendril", indicating the tender, cautious nature of the developmental strivings. Both these forward and trailing elements, reflecting the repetition of old behavioural or emotional patterns, may be embedded in any communication, and, in particular, the dream.

Illustrating this approach, Livingston (2001) reports a dream in which a dreamer was frightened by a large "gross" roach that he was unable to kill. He said that even though the bug's head "started to look like a kitten's head ... I wanted to wake up to get out of there because the bug wouldn't die" (p. 21). After exploring some of the frightening, ugly, and disgusting parts of the dream, another member noted the appearance of the kitten's head. This intervention shifted the discussion away from the repetitive bad, ugly aspects of the dreamer's self to the gentler, sweeter aspects of self, representing the forward edge. Following reflection on the emergence of the kitten's head, the group focused on the transformation taking place in the dreamer and identified other personal transformations. This material was followed by a woman presenting a sexual dream, experienced as shameful, but facilitating her exploration of previously unexamined and frightening sectors of herself.

Identification of positive (forward edge) change could be interpreted as a flight from further examination of destructive and ugly self percepts. In this example, however, the consequence was that another member could report a dream which brought to the fore previously warded off sectors of self. The sequence suggests that a forward edge focus can serve a mirroring selfobject function, strengthening the therapeutic alliance and thus facilitating the patient's or group's exploration of deeper, trailing edge self issues. From the group self perspective the forward edge focus strengthens the group ideal of appreciating the potential of each member.

An advantage of reporting dreams in groups is the presence and availability of peers. Members, with the interpretative assistance of the therapist, soon learn that a dream is not only a personal statement about the dreamer but contains aspects of the group culture and discourse. In situations where the dreamer is unable to meaningfully associate to his/her own dream, members can bring their own associations to the fore. These may be either to affects, main elements, fragments, or aspects of the dream sequence portraying dynamic processes within the group. As illustrated by the above example, members may learn how to comment about the dream elements and the process as portrayed by the dream. This is a crucial ability for a well-functioning analytic group self.

Our work with dreams in groups is not prescriptive. Whatever is said is heard by everyone, and this is particularly true for the therapist's utterances. Thus, an intervention or exploration of a dream focusing on the dreamer is heard and experienced by all present. Others' responses may include a sense of the therapist as an enhancing selfobject or as a destructive, disruptive force. Interpretations of the dream as reflecting group-as-a-whole processes almost certainly will not be completely accurate and could narcissistically injure one or more members. By monitoring the process after each intervention, therapists can learn a good deal about injured individuals' self-stabilizing responses. Fosshage (2002) notes that selfobject responsiveness through the life cycle serves to modify prior self-organization and promotes growth. He asserts that without such experiences, one would be stuck with the relational patterns formed in early childhood. Peer and therapist exploration of dreams serve as a template of selfobject responsiveness and add to the evolving group culture, which values attachments, self-reflection, and the understanding of others as having their own minds and perspectives.

Stem et al. (1998) have emphasised the importance of both conscious and unconscious "relational learning" that contributes to change. Of particular significance is the "moment of meeting" which reflects authentic, deeply felt personal contact. Member-to-member or therapist-to-member experiences in working to understand a dream, not only for the dreamer but for all present, may provide such moments. These intensely experienced moments are likely to increase members' capacity to manage affects and to see and appreciate others as subjects in contrast to objects primarily used to fulfil one's needs.

Fonagy, Gergely, Jurist, and Target (2002) highlight an additional developmental task that could be facilitated by empathic exploration of dreams. This work can help shift psychic equivalence thinking (characterised by the equation of the internal with the external) to self-reflective functioning (thinking that demonstrates understanding of others' internal wishes and emotions). Empathic responsiveness to the dream, either from therapist or a group member, may provide the moment of meeting, thereby deepening the dialogue.

In the following two illustrations we demonstrate how the dream can be an effective communication and how the work within the group can mediate between the individual and the group-as-a-whole, thereby contributing both to individual development (self-reflective and representational functioning) and an unblocking of an arrested group self.

Clinical examples

The sexual assault

Jim's behaviour toward Irene was perceived by several of the other female group members as thinly veiled sexual solicitations and in several sessions, they expressed their annoyance with him. The men, and in particular Frank, whose characteristic defence was distancing, resisted becoming involved. It was in this context that Frank reported a dream:

> There is a man who copulates with a woman. Thereafter it is my turn. However, I discover that her genitals are poorly developed. I can't get it in. It all happened on a veranda. Then somebody knocks on the door. I believe there are several men coming to rape her, and I flee down the gutter. Halfway down I change my mind and climb up again. On the veranda I find several men and women sitting there and talking to each other.

Frank's associations quickly turned to an incident when he was 10 years old. His 15-year-old brother and several friends had tried to seduce, if not rape, his 12-year-old sister. She had barely escaped. He was a passive, excitedly stimulated, and upset witness who subsequently became highly self-critical for not intervening. As he told the story, Frank became increasingly angry, primarily at his brother, but also at himself for his cowardice. Jim's seductive behaviour, highlighted by the women, had reminded Frank of his brother's attempted seduction. He could not involve himself now, just as he was unable to intervene then. The group readily grasped the connection between Frank's childhood story and his anger and shame in the here-and-now.

The therapist noted that not much had been said about the last part of the dream. He suggested:

> There is a crucial difference between then and now. In childhood Frank had no one to speak to about this shameful experience. But in the dream, he finds 'several men and women sitting together and talking on the veranda. I wonder if this might signify the opportunity to talk with people in the group'.

Although Frank feared fighting with the symbolic brother and being condemned for his own sexual desire in the dream, he was able to return to the "veranda." The benign presence of talking adults, absent in his childhood, now enabled him to approach anew this part of his past and acquire a new perspective on himself and his group experiences.

We think of this dream as being stimulated by a conflict in the group self, a tension concerning what rules of discourse should reign. These rules include a "pretend mode" wherein reality may be distorted by acting on it in playful ways (Fonagy et al., 2002, p. 57). The pretend mode is not real in the same sense as ordinary social reality. Pretend mode discourse is necessary in analytic groups in order to establish the sense of safety necessary for members to experience and express shameful ways of thinking, feeling and behaving. The presence of the pretend mode is marked, that is, signalled in some nonverbal manner.

Jim had claimed that he had done nothing more than follow the group norm by speaking about what was on his mind. He asked, "Are sexual feelings taboo in this group?" The women responded that it was the way he talked about sexual feelings, that it was not reflective, but rather abusive and exploitative. They experienced him as enacting his lust, and further accused him of not marking his speech and transgressing the established pretend mode of the group discourse (Austin, 1962), of displaying his raw and undigested sexual lust for the sake of gratification, not reflection.

Taking sides in this conflict is not our task as therapists. There might well have been elements of "gratification" in Jim's approach toward Irene, but these elements were surely augmented by the women. When the conflict escalated, it soon reached a level of projective identification where heated mutual accusations dominated the scene at the expense of reflective functioning. Under these circumstances, the group self was temporarily suffused by psychic equivalence thinking. The result was loss of the ordinary, more playful discourse.

Fonagy et al. (2002) assert that playing in situations governed by mature adults facilitates the transformation of psychic equivalent thinking to representational thinking. The traumatic childhood incident which Frank recalled was an episode where the boundaries of the pretend mode of play were lost. What started as a (sex ual) play, had escalated and turned into a near nightmare of non-play realities. For Frank the episode had model scene qualities in which specific transactions trigger core affect laden responses within the individual or group (Correale & Celli, 1998; Lichtenberg, Lachmann, & Fosshage, 1992). He had established characterological defences which placed him in uninvolved positions vis-a-vis his surrounds. He became a lonely onlooker; to become more involved might threaten his capacity to contain or cope with his emotional responses. He lacked the experience of playing with dangerous ideas and feelings in the presence of a benign grown-up who could monitor the boundaries. The group self dynamics came to resemble the nightmare in his unconscious. Seemingly innocent and playful impulses could turn to threatening realities.

The therapist's interpretation at the end of this sequence served didactic purposes. By equating those sitting on the veranda with the group members, he brought into greater awareness for both Frank and the others the group selfobject function; that is, the experience of being in the group as a safe, responsive venue, a prerequisite for exploring frightful fantasies. For Frank, the group was a contrast to what he had missed in his childhood. By highlighting the veranda group, with its differentiated members talking to each other and exchanging ideas, the therapist focused on the dreamer's hope for a new experience, in essence the forward edge (Tolpin, 2002). The ensemble imago contained a feeling of positive surprise and a wish for belonging.

While there is an ongoing debate in the literature regarding the role of insight versus (new) relational experience (Fosshage, 2002), this clinical example illuminates how a new relational experience (the selfobject function of the group) can facilitate self-understanding (insight). The new self-understanding, in turn, had profound effects on the further treatment course, providing new perspectives for the working through of pathogenic complexes in the structure of the self.

The playing group

Mary told the following dream: *"I am in a conference hall where somebody is giving a talk on a serious matter. Beside me sits Allen [another group member]. We link together and swing from side to side. We have fun, smile and laugh."* The dream quickly became linked to an important theme in Mary's life. She was a dutiful woman, deeply engaged in professional and societal issues, at the expense of other aspects of her life. An important theme for Mary had been how she could lead a more joyful life. In the dream, Allen came to represent a bridge to this goal. He would serve as a model for having fun, thereby expanding Mary's restricted sense of self, through a twinship selfobject transference. The group explored these themes of self-sacrifice and wish to play for an extended period. The therapist found no reason to intervene, although he noted that the group had not commented on the theme of rebellion, as in the turning from the serious discourse of the conference to play and fun. During the following discussion Allen was unusually active and assertive. He was obviously vitalised by his role in Mary's dream.

After a while, the therapist acknowledged Allen's level of activity, which he linked to a dream Allen had told in the previous meeting. In that dream, which had been given an Oedipal interpretation, Allen owned a more impressive mobile phone than the therapist. The therapist suggested that Allen, who had been rather inhibited in the group, now seemed to be in touch with a more assertive part of himself. For Allen, activity had been associated with a dangerous rivalry with the therapist. It seemed as if that were no longer the case. Noting that in the previous dream Allen used his mobile phone to call a woman, the therapist, continuing his lengthy interpretation, observed that it was as if Mary had understood the unconscious (but interpreted) message in Allen's dream. Her own Oedipal conflict involved a need to satisfy her father's claim for serious work on important societal issues and renounce sexual explorative play with peers. Allen, who now dared to challenge the therapist in a sexual arena, seemed to confirm for Mary some of her own suppressed sexual and joyful desires. Through this affirmation, she too could dare to rebel against the deadly serious father/ therapist. In order to justify the last element in the interpretation, the therapist reminded Mary of her experience several months previously when she had attended the therapist's lecture at a professional meeting. Following this extended interpretation, the group immersed itself in further associations to the themes in these dreams.

These dreams occurred in a well-functioning, long-term analytic group. They emerged from the matrix of an advanced group self unhampered by any conflicts suffused by projective identifications. The group self was characterised by a well-established pretend mode which provided the members freedom to play with "dangerous things".

In our opinion, a sophisticated group self has integrated at least some notion of social unconscious processes, in which the members influence each other and influence the group-self. While the reality of the unconscious cannot be proved, its effects can be demonstrated through the interplay between the observable here-and-now and the dream narratives. In this instance the therapist spelled out how Mary's and Allen's Oedipal conflicts intermingled, involved the therapist, were portrayed in the dreams, and played out in the theatre of the group. The therapist's intervention represented an affirmation (mirroring) of forward edge work of both patients. Both were exploring the possibility of new, more assertive behaviours.

Discussion

In *The Impossible Profession,* Janet Malcolm (1981) describes the clinician's task as maintaining multiple perspectives and not prematurely foreclosing potentially productive avenues for understanding therapeutic communication. Harwood (2002) lists seven differing perspectives in which she might examine dreams. Group therapists may be severely challenged in this respect because any dream may communicate at multiple levels. Dreams, presented in group psychotherapy, are events in which the dreamer is trying to communicate to the self and others in the group about the self, other, self-with-other, group processes, and/ or the larger environment, including the more general culture. It may refer to the past, present, or future. The manifest dream imagery is no longer seen as only a representation of a disguised wish. Rather it may be viewed as a metaphor, or representation of the dreamer's current concerns. It is not the dream itself that is therapeutic, but the subsequent responses which may amplify and solidify the members' self or the group self. In our illustrations we have attempted to exemplify these notions.

In our first vignette, Frank, stimulated by the sexuality embedded in the group transactions, brought forth a dream which addressed his conflict in the present over his passivity and shame. The undisguised nature of his sexual failure and his flight only to return to a place where gentle conversation was occurring all signal perceptions of the group that potentially can serve his developmental progressive thrust. The second vignette communicates Mary's sense of having increased ability to play even in the context of "serious matters." In these examples from long-term treatment, a group setting is overtly represented in one dream, and a specific group member is incorporated into the second dream, both seeming to suggest that the group was experienced as a sufficiently safe setting in which growth and change could take place.

Certainly, the value of any group dream is its communication both to the dreamer and others. How and in what manner the therapist and the other members respond in order to take advantage of the opportunity is multi-determined. The thrust of this paper has been to illustrate the patients' presentation of dreams in an effort to communicate about difficulties within the group setting that have interfered with their effective use of the group, and how this served as a stimulus for change in a growth enhancing direction.

References

Atwood, G. E. & Stolorow, R. D. (1984). *Structures of Subjectivity: Explorations in Psychoanalytic Phenomenology.* New York: The Analytic Press.

Austin, J. L. (1962). *How to Do Things with Words.* Oxford: Oxford University Press.

Bacal, H. A. (1985). Optimal responsiveness and the therapeutic process. In A. Goldberg (Ed.), *Progress in Seif Psychology, vol 1* (pp. 202–226). New York: Guilford.

Correale, A. & Celli, A. M. (1998). The model-scene in group psycho therapy with chronic psychotic patients. *International Journal of Group Psychotherapy,* 48: 55–68.

Fonagy, P., Gergely, G., Jurist, E. L. & Target, M. (2002). *Affect Regulation, Mentalization, and the Development of the Seif.* New York: Other Press.

Fosshage, J. L. (1997). The organizing function of dream mentation. *Con temporary Psychoanalysis,* 33: 429–458.

Fosshage, J. L. (2002). Love and anger within the analytic relationship: A Clinical workshop. Paper presented at the International Conference on the Psychology of the Self, Washington, DC.

Freud, S. (1900). The interpretation of dreams. In J. Strachey (Ed. and trans.), *The Standard Edition of the Complete Psychological Works of Sigmund Freud* (Vol. 6, pp. 1–627). London: Hogarth Press.

Harwood, I. (2002). Discussion of Martin Livingston's working playspace. In C. Neri, M. Pines, & R. Friedman (Eds.), *Dreams Ingroup Psychotherapy: Theory and Technique* (pp. 191–196). London: Jessica Kingsley.

Harwood, I. N. H. (1998). Advances in group psychotherapy and self psychology: An intersubjective approach. In I. Harwood & M. Pines (Eds.), *Seif Experiences in Group: Intersubjective and Seif Psychological Path Ways to Human Understanding* (pp. 30–46). London: Jessica Kingsley.

Karterud, S. (1992). Group dreams revisited. *Group Analysis,* 25: 207–221.

Karterud, S. & Stone, W. N. (2003). The group self: A neglected aspect of group psychotherapy. *Group Analysis,* 36: 7–22.

Karterud, S. W. (1998). The group self, empathy, intersubjectivity and hermeneutics: A group analytic perspective. In I. Harwood & M. Pines (Eds.), *Self Experiences in Group: Intersubjective and Seif Psychological Pathways to Human Understanding* (pp. 83–98). London: Jessica Kingsley.

Kohut, H. (1976). Creativeness, charisma, group psychology: Reflections on Freud's seif analysis. In J. E. Gedo & G. H. Pollock (Eds.), *Freud: The Fusion of Science and Humanism.* New York: International Universities Press.

Kohut, H. (1984). *How Does Analysis Cure?* Chicago: University of Chicago Press.

Lichtenberg, J. D., Lachmann, F. M. & Fosshage, J. L. (1992). *Seif and Motivational Systems: Toward a Theory of Psychoanalytic Technique.* Hillsdale: The Analytic Press.

Livingston, M. S. (2001). Self psychology, dreams and group psychotherapy: Working in the playspace. *Group,* 25: 15–26.

Malcolm, J. (1981). *Psychoanalysis: The Impossible Profession.* Northvale: Jason Aronson.

Ornstein, P. H. (1987). On self-state dreams in psychoanalytic treatment process. In A. Rothstein (Ed.), *The Interpretation of Dreams in Clinical Work* (pp. 87–104). Madison: International Universities Press.

Stem, N. D., Sander, L. W., Nahum, J. P., Harrison, A. M., Lyons-Ruth, K., Morgan, A. C., et al. (1998). Non-interpretive mechanisms in psycho analytic therapy: The 'something more' than interpretation. *International Journal of Psycho-Analysis*, 79: 903–921.

Stone, W. N. (1992). The clinical application of self psychology. In R. H. Klein, H. S. Bernard, & D. L. Singer (Eds.), *Handbook of Contemporary Group Psychotherapy: Contributions from Object Relations, Seif Psychology and Social Systems Theories* (pp. 177–208). Madison: International Universities Press.

Stone, W. N. & Whitman, R. M. (1977). Contribution of the psychology of the seif to group process and group therapy. *International Journal of Group Psychotherapy*, 27: 343–359.

Tolpin, M. (2002). Doing psychoanalysis of normal development: Forward edge transferences. In A. Goldberg (Ed.), *Postmodern Seif Psychology: Progress in Seif Psychology* (pp. 167–190). Hillsdale: Analytic Press.

Chapter 4

Constructing and mentalizing the matrix

Sigmund Karterud

Abstract

This text was presented as the S. H. Foulkes memorial lecture in London 2012. Here I describe the empirical process that accompanied the evolution of mentalization-based group therapy. It did not come out of the blue. During the years around the Millenium shift, my research group did a lot of experimentation and empirical studies on group analytic therapies with personality-disordered clients, naturalistic as well as a randomised controlled study, and compared our results to other international studies. When we finally adopted the mentalizing model, it was still an experiment, later to be confirmed by research evidence. Most notably, it was conducted and accompanied by manuals and adherence scales. This work impacted our notion about the group matrix concept. In this article I emphasise an evolutionary perspective that acknowledge the existence of group matrices among other mammals, in particular among the great apes, but uphold their inability to mentalize the matrix. I maintain that Homo sapiens were able to mentalize the matrix, in contrast to the great apes that failed in mentalizing it and had to live in it in a situation-bound manner. Mentalizing the matrix implies being able to construct collective meaningful narratives and histories as explanations for things being as they are with the individuals, their transactions and the group. It has implied storytellers, writers, libraries and other storehouses of cultural capital, and eventually the Internet that unites "the global village". It is maintained that matrix refers to a structure that unites and differentiate groups. Therapists co-construct therapeutic group structures. This task has been somewhat neglected in group analytic theory, as if the group matrix develops "out of itself". Finally, there is a discussion of the implications as to constructing group matrices that suit the containment and developmental needs of e.g., borderline patients.

S. H. Foulkes coined the central concepts of group analysis (Foulkes, 1948, 1957). Among them is the concept of matrix, which is the theme of tonight's lecture, and now in concert with the more modern concept of mentalization. Both of these concepts are embedded in rich theoretical networks (Karterud, 1999; Fonagy et al.,

DOI: 10.4324/9781003625810-4

2003). Without the matrix concept, I believe the theory of group analysis would collapse. In Foulkes' terminology, the concept of matrix refers to the established communicational web or network that exists among people who are united for some purpose (Foulkes, 1973). He distinguished between the foundation matrix and the dynamic matrix. The foundation matrix refers to that part of the communicational network that stems from our common biological makeup, our senses, our capacity for linguistic communication, our particular brand of language and culture, and, we must add, our capacity for mentalizing. The dynamic matrix refers to the ongoing and fluctuating communicational network in a particular group.

Both the foundation and the dynamic matrix precede the concept of mentalization in a historical sense. Foulkes himself pointed to the evolutionary roots of the matrix. When people join groups, he said, they are affected by 'ancient tribal feelings' (Foulkes, 1957: p. 235). In evolution, tribes are a rather recent occurrence. In fact, we see concerted group behaviour even among unicellular organisms, like the bacteria. Not to mention the social insects. The capacity of individuals to communicate and perform united actions according to certain patterns, does not presuppose any mind. The first group matrices to be formed on earth were thus rather simple. When mind appeared, around 550 million years ago, group matrices became more dynamic and sophisticated. Equipped with a mind, the animal had an internal working space, which could delay immediate action and permit negotiations with other agents in the world. When we come to our close relatives, the great apes, we find quite sophisticated groups with established communicational patterns, membership rules and social hierarchies. Life in such communities is tough. In their natural habitats these animals are stressed, actually with intermittent high cortisol levels, due to predators, internal rivals, external rivalries from other troops, scarcity of food, natural disasters, and the like. Although the great apes have minds, as well as emotions and feelings, and the ability to interpret each other to some limited sense in the here and now, and to live in rather large groups, they have stagnated and are by now at the brink of extinction.

Some few individuals broke off, by some lucky mutations around six million years ago. A small group of their descendants, possibly not more than a hundred individuals in the first wave, left Africa some 60-70,000 years ago, and Homo sapiens now count around seven billion people. The main reason for this amazing reproductive success was most probably the capacity for implicit as well as explicit mentalization, a capacity that evolved, in concert with language, probably sometime during the last 100,000 years (Corballis, 2007). Due to this capacity, Homo sapiens have been able to mentalize the matrix, in contrast to the great apes that failed in mentalizing it but had to live in it in a situation-bound manner (Bogdan, 2000). By mentalizing the matrix, I mean constructing a collective meaningful narrative and history as explanations for things being as they are with the individuals, their transactions and the group. Storytellers appeared, then writers, libraries and other storehouses of cultural capital, and eventually the Internet that unites "the global village".

Foulkes described the individual as a "nodal point" in the matrix (Foulkes, 1948). This metaphor conveys images of the individuals as small particles in a vast terrain, and images of the formidable group forces, for good or for worse that pass right through the individual, "through his very core", as Foulkes liked to express himself. In a therapeutic group the pathogenic experiences of the individual, formerly not being communicated verbally, might find resonance through another mind and enter into a group associative communicational spiral that helps the individual to symbolise the unsymbolised and express the formerly inexpressible. This part of Foulkes' theory is remarkably modern. However, like all psychoanalysts at his time, he lacked a proper theory of emotions. Thus, the metaphors of the matrix and the individuals as the nodal points need to be complemented with modern theories.

Since Foulkes there has been an enormous growth in our knowledge about intersubjectivity and emotions. Intersubjectivity is the foundation of the human self (Karterud, 1998). This has been the guiding idea of continental philosophers since the early work of Husserl, through Heidegger, Sartre, Gadamer and Ricoeur. The slogan "being thrown into the world" (Heidegger, 1927) and Ricoeur's title *Oneself as Another* (1992) attest to this ontogenic fate. Without being minded by the mind of another, the self will not develop its innate capacity for mentalization. This claim started as a philosophical idea. In our times it is explored by "hard science".

In the first place, that which is being minded is the organism's emotional response to events in the surrounds and in his/her body. Nowadays we talk about *primary emotional systems* that are innate action programmes, which can be experienced as feelings. There is yet no consensus on *which* emotional systems that are primary. Personally, I vote for Jaak Panksepp's seven candidates: *Exploration/curiosity, fear, separation distress, anger, lust, care and play/joy.* These emotions are found among most mammals, as well as their corresponding feeling states (Panksepp, 1998). We know much about the neurobiology of these emotions and their brain localization, as well as their ability of being triggered by mirror neurons. It is a plausible hypothesis that the contagious nature of emotions, their tendency to rapidly spread through the matrix and lighten up the individual nodal points, so to speak, is contingent upon the mirror neuron system (Iacobini & Mazziotta, 2007). However, we also know that there are vast differences between individuals with respect to their emotional reactivity, emotion awareness, emotion tolerance, emotional self-understanding, and emotional expressivity. Typical differences are found between the different personality prototypes, some being more inert while others being highly reactive (Karterud, Wilberg, & Urnes, 2010). Does it matter then to the group matrix how the individuals in the nodal points are designed with respect to basic personality features?

As for therapeutic groups, Foulkes was, as we know, remarkably optimistic on behalf of the group and its matrix. It did not matter that much, he said, how groups are composed with respect to individuals, since they will deviate from the norms that constitute healthy groups in highly individual ways, due to their different life experiences. As a group the individuals will compensate for each other's

than what is reported in most studies of individual psychotherapy for borderline patients (Bateman & Fonagy, 1999; 2001; 2009; Giessen-Bloo, 2006; Leichsenring & Rabung, 2008; Perry et al., 1999).

On the top of this we found some discouraging results in a randomised clinical trial at our department, comparing day hospital and subsequent conjoint group-individual psychotherapy with individual eclectic psychotherapy conducted by private practitioners for a range of personality disorders (n = 113). A three year follow up showed the outcome was pretty alike for conjoint therapy compared to individual psychotherapy, except for global functioning, measured by the GAF, where individual psychotherapy did significantly better (Gullestad et al., 2012). Also here, the effect sizes were small for the group psychotherapy phase that followed day hospital treatment. Moreover, we recently found that *when we split the patients with respect to their level of mentalizing, measured according to reflective functioning (RF) based upon Adult Attachment Interviews, the patients who had the lowest RF responded very well to individual psychotherapy, but poorly to the combined group-individual therapy* (Gullestad et al., 2013). In contrast, patients with higher RF (>3) responded equally well to both treatment conditions. This is the first time it has been demonstrated that patients with low mentalizing capacity respond differently to different treatment conditions.

How did we interpret these results? Since there were no differences between presumably high qualified group therapists and less qualified, *it seems that the group dynamics take precedence over the impact of the therapists.* Or stated differently, as long as one conducts along the principles of free group association in groups with severe personality disorder, the resulting group dynamic seems to take its own course and the group therapist's ability to influence it seems minimal. This does not need to be a concern if the group dynamic promotes self-integration and self-development among the members. However, the results from the RCT *indicate that the group dynamic might impede development for patients with low mentalizing capacity rather than promoting it.* The kind of dynamic in those groups may become overwhelming in some way for the more poorly functioning patients.

If these speculations are right, they may be disappointing from a group analytic point of view. However, they are not so surprising in the light of recent research data on the neurobiology of borderline patients (Siever & Weinstein 2009). It has consistently been shown that borderline patients are more sensitive, which means having a lower threshold for emotional reaction than normal controls, and that they react more intensely. In addition, it has been shown, that even in safe test situations, they are more aroused than normal controls. Data from a recent game experiment shows that borderline patients display less trust and cooperativeness than normal controls, and by this tend to be less successful in social situations (King-Casas et al., 2008). In fact, they tend to lose money as well as friends and have a tendency to become hyper-aroused and lose their mentalizing capacity.

Gather eight such individuals in a room, all of them very sensitive, aroused at the outset, distrustful, having trouble cooperating successfully with others, easily losing their mentalizing capacity – it is not surprising that the odds are low for the development of a warm, caring, mutually supporting group that is curious about exploring mental states. However, it is important to underline that patients in the borderline range do vary considerably with respect to their mentalizing capacity. Given a turbulent group, it seems that patients with a moderately reduced mentalizing capacity might benefit from group interaction, while patients with a lower (RF<3) capacity find it harder to integrate their experiences in a way that promote self-development.

One of the most curious facts in this field is the large variation in outcome. We recently conducted a five-year follow up study for symptom distress on 770 patients (mostly personality disorders) in our treatment research network (Kvarstein & Karterud, 2013). 43% of these 770 patients received group psychotherapy after day hospital treatment. When we looked at symptom distress in the five-year follow up, there was a huge variance. 47% displayed reliable change and did very well. Most of them were almost symptom free. However, the 36% that experienced no reliable change were still symptomatically very disturbed.

How can we account for these differences? Attending group psychotherapy, had little impact upon the course. However, there was an interaction between personality and group psychotherapy. Having borderline PD *and* attending long-term group psychotherapy made a significant positive contribution. Borderline patients *do* change for the better, but to a lesser degree than we would expect when we look at the results from other therapies. There seem to be important differences between different categories of personality disorder.

The kind of patients that respond the least to this kind of group treatment were actually patients with severe avoidant PD. They are even more frightened in groups than borderline patients and resort to avoidant strategies, which are hard to challenge in free associative groups. Nevertheless, it is hard to predict the long-term course. Patients with the same personality diagnoses and about the same level of functioning may have a quite different long-term course. Our best models explain between 35% and 50% of the variance in different outcome measures. There is reason to believe that if we had added mentalizing capacity and some quality measurement of the treatment, the explained variance would have increased.

It took us a long time to realise that the measured outcome of our treatment was somewhat lower than what several competing therapies were reporting. Was it the same for the other units in our research network? We compared our data with data from the group therapies at 15 similar units. The results were about the same. Group psychotherapy yielded a significant positive change, but to a modest degree. The Department of Personality Psychiatry at Oslo University Hospital included a day hospital programme and an outpatient unit that contained around 12 groups. We also had a research unit and there was an expectation of contributing to the development of knowledge and technologies in the field of mental health.

From a purely clinical point of view, we could have survived some more years with "ordinary", but modest treatment results. However, from a research point of view, it seemed that we had reached a dead end. There was no more energy, so to speak, no vitality and creativity in sight within the tradition we used to work, i.e., the tradition of therapeutic communities, day hospitals and "traditional" group analytic psychotherapy for patients with personality disorders.

This perception is an interesting phenomenon in itself. Was this a local phenomenon, a sign of burn-out, or did it reflect more profound changes that were occurring in the society at large and in our profession? Unfortunately, I cannot explore this topic here. The short story is that our department, after lengthy discussions, decided to implement mentalization-based treatment (MBT). All in all, MBT was rather close, albeit distinctly different. Above all, the efficiency of the model had been documented, but the freshness of the ideas was important as well, the new theory of borderline PD, the embeddedness of the theory in modern theories of evolution, neurobiology and child development, and a close link between the theory of psychopathology and the rationale for specific therapeutic interventions.

We implemented the intensive outpatient version of MBT in August 2008 and closed down our day hospital. Paradoxical some might say, since the isolated effect of the day hospital part was rather good. It was the continuation group psychotherapy that was the problem.

However, if one aims at longer term treatment, it is a bad choice to start with 18 weeks short term day hospital treatment, and then make changes with groups and therapists. For a long time, we had disliked this practice from an attachment point of view.

Our first task then, as a highly group-oriented department, was to reorient our therapists and train and support them in individual MBT, since MBT is a conjoint group-individual treatment. This training was facilitated by our development, in cooperation with Anthony Bateman, of the MBT adherence and competence scale for individual psychotherapy (Karterud & Bateman, 2010). It took us several rounds of discussions with Bateman and other Nordic colleagues, and we tested several versions of this scale. However, it was not that complicated since it built upon a rich literature by Bateman and Fonagy (2004, 2006).

In a recent reliability study, we have shown that it is possible to rate therapists as to which degree they comply with the mentalization-based mode of treatment (Karterud et al., 2013). This manual has been very helpful in training and supervising staff.

The group therapy component of MBT turned out to be a harder nut. Previous literature contained fewer concrete recommendations. We realised once more that group psychotherapy is a far more complex and challenging task than individual psychotherapy. We started by implementing more of the techniques from individual MBT and studied the results on video recordings for a considerable period. Overall, the group dynamics became possibly a bit more productive and less harmful, but we witnessed no revolution.

At a certain point we realised that we had nothing to lose from embarking upon a more radical experiment. We had always been loyal to the basic tenets of group analysis. What if we killed several of our darlings and started afresh with a new design based upon the theory of mentalization and its pathologies for borderline patients? How would the groups look then?

If we define group analysis as a general theory of man as a social being, and group analytic psychotherapy as a clinical application for more well-functioning individuals, where should we place mentalization-based group therapy? As a discipline "under" group analytic psychotherapy, or "beside it"? The metaphors of under and besides, as I use them here, convey some important implications.

As a discipline under group analytic psychotherapy, it would imply that it should retain the basic ingredients, among which is the principle of free group association. If we define it as besides, we are more freed from the canonic ingredients of group analytic psychotherapy. We are so used to free group association that we, within the realm of psychodynamic group psychotherapy, seldom question its validity.

Historically speaking, the principle of free group association was derived from the principle of free association in psychoanalysis. In psychoanalysis it was developed as a technique to deal with the defence mechanism that Freud initially regarded as the prototype of defence mechanisms: Repression. Free association loosens up the barrier between the conscious and the unconscious, and makes repressed thoughts and affects come closer to the conscious mind.

However, it is a long time since someone has claimed that borderline patients suffer from repression. When they are more frightened and aroused at the outset of the group, it is probably due to multiple causes—which end up in the final, common pathway of poor emotion regulation. So why should free group association be the answer? Why should the group therapist just sit down and wait and see what happens and try at his/her best to mentalize what is in the matrix?

The alternative to free group association can be formulated as *constructing the matrix*, which means that the therapist takes control of the group by structuring it in a certain way so as to favour certain processes and inhibit others. Being in the position to design a kind of group therapy from scratch, we asked ourselves: What should be the guiding principles of this group construction, and are they amenable to borderline patients? Paraphrasing Foulkes' formulation of the group as an arena for "ego training in action", we adopt the slogan of Anthony Bateman that the group is a "training arena for mentalization". How do we construct such a training ground for the enhancement of the mentalizing capabilities of very vulnerable members?

Firstly, by being more explicit to group members regarding the aim of the group, and what is expected from them. By this new approach we explicitly state that group members are expected to bring to the group difficult interpersonal encounters, and that everybody should try to engage in an exploration of such encounters by a mentalizing stance. What this means is discussed *in the psychoeducational group, which the members attend parallel to the dynamic group during the first three months.* Moreover, we advise group therapists to:

1. Discuss the group more profoundly between the sessions.
2. Take hold of the opening phase of the group.
3. Install open reflection on the process during the last third part of the group.
4. Invite what we label "balanced mentalizing turn-taking".
5. Oscillate between external and internal interpersonal events.
6. Stop destructive emotional escalations.
7. Engage the group members in exploration of events.
8. Keep an open, mindful dialogue with the co-therapist around how to understand the here and now.
9. Refrain from complicated metaphors and interpretations that suggest that the therapists know "what really is going on" in the group.

I will elaborate some of these points to explain the underlying ideas further:

1) *Poor group cohesion* is a great problem in these groups since they are composed of individuals with poor self-cohesion, which has negative consequences in its own right. Poor group cohesion increases the risk of dropout, and it undermines the morale of the group. It also impedes attachment. Accordingly, we advocate that the therapists "build bridges" between the group sessions, *by starting the group* with references to the last meeting, mentioning all members and suggesting some implications for the forthcoming meeting. This intervention is believed to strengthen group cohesion, by "*minding the group*", as well as *strengthening the members' experience of being minded.* The therapists actually say: This is what we have thought about the group and its members since the last group meeting. It is delivered in a manner that invites comments and dialogue, and it is also supposed to *stimulate metacognition* by inviting a reflection on what this immediate past means for the upcoming future:

   E.g., In the light of previous meetings and what we have heard about your current concerns, how should we proceed from here? Did Anna finish her stuff last time? What has happened to Greg in the meantime? Then something happened towards the end of the session, and it has been a long time since we have heard about you, Peter, and you, Helena. And there might be other things . . .
2) As I have already mentioned, this approach implies some degree of *turn-taking.* Turn-taking is a despised word (and practice) among psychodynamic group therapists. However, we would like to restore its respectability, while realizing that we are playing with psychological fire here. We will introduce the concept "*balanced mentalizing turn-taking*". The word balanced refers to the group and means that the group therapists take active measures to bring the imbalance in the group, with respect to time and attention, up for reflection. It says to the monopoliser that perhaps you have had your share for some time, and to the silent member, that perhaps you should enter the stage. I say "perhaps" here, since the group therapists do not impose, but suggest and try to make the obvious group dynamics open for reflection. The structure we propose does

not promote turn-taking for its own sake, as a matter of justice, as an equal share to everybody. It promotes turn-taking as *a means to work with interpersonal events.* Poor mentalization has many manifestations. The one that lends itself best for exploration in a group therapeutic situation, is the interpersonal encounter. Besides, we know that mentalizing in close relations is a major difficulty for borderline patients. Accordingly, we invite turn-taking where the focus is on some kind of troublesome interpersonal encounter from the previous week, either remembered from the past, experienced in the present or anticipated for the future.

3) The primary task of the therapists during such turn-taking is to *help the group to mentalize the event.* This involves the very capacity to construct a narrative that gives coherence, context and meaning to the event, as well as the capacity to identify the mentalization problems inherent in the narrative and to explore their significance. Turn-taking is not a means for individual therapy in groups. *It is about creating scenes that the members can explore.*
4) Being involved in such a task, there will inevitably occur what might be labelled *interpersonal events in the here and now.* Some kind of emotional reaction will emerge between the members, and the group will face the challenge of exploring similar events as those reported and do the mentalizing work as it happens in the here and now. To assist properly in this task, the therapists should employ the techniques which we have outlined in the MBT manual: the not knowing stance, curious exploration, regulating the emotional arousal, adjusting to the current level of mentalizing, having an affect focus, stop and rewind, deal with psychic equivalence phenomena, etc.
5) The skilful therapists should help the group to oscillate between outside group events, events in the here and now, and stimulate metacognitive reflections on the group level. I have already mentioned the introductory metacognitive invitation. Other comments might be: "How are we doing?", "Did we understand what was going on?", "Are we approaching a closure of this sequence? How is it, have you learned something, Eric, from this discussion?", And "I must remind you that there are 20 minutes left. We have this unresolved business with Greg and Lena, Ann has asked for some space and then we have the events that you must face, Peter. What do we do?"

The structure that I have outlined incorporates the therapeutic stance as it is practiced in most of the current MBT programmes. It does not do away with splitting, projective identification, mental blocks, withdrawal, emotional explosions, lack of motivation and other not so pleasant group phenomena. However, clinical experiences suggest that it makes those phenomena more manageable for therapeutic transformations in groups. What are the costs? I have not emphasised previously that the therapists are rather active. Much more active than what is considered appropriate for group analysis. But how is the effect of that on the group level? We know that there is a danger that active group therapists might create passive dependent patients. However, we try to counteract it by different means.

Firstly, by rapidly introducing group level metacognitive questions. Secondly, by being careful not to do the mentalizing work on behalf of the patients. Thirdly, by being very cautious with interpretations that suggest that the therapists have a special kind of insight into the unconscious realm of the individuals and the group. We suggest that the phantasy of the omnipotence of the therapists, coupled with "envious attacks on linking" is an intersubjective phenomenon. If the therapists actually behave in an omnipotent way, they may well stimulate envy and a corresponding self-state of being helpless and deprived. The stance we advocate for the therapists is the opposite. It is engaged, open-minded, curious, relatively transparent (e.g., actively exploring one's own contribution to the ongoing transactions), and above all genuinely "not knowing", but with a curious interest in "finding out together". By these means it is not our experience that we create dependency groups.

Besides what has been published by Bateman and Fonagy (1999, 2001, 2009), do we have any indications that mentalization-based group therapy works for the better also in contexts like ours? We do not know for sure since this is work in progress and since MBT is a conjoint treatment. However, at our department we monitor the clinical work through the research unit. The preliminary results from our outpatient unit are good. Until April 2009, 23 patients had terminated the MBT programme. The data so far indicates a stronger and more rapid treatment effect compared to the old programme. Anyhow, the preliminary results represent an encouragement to proceed.

How might we eventually prove that this kind of group therapy for borderline patients is better than unstructured free associative groups? If this really is the case, and if we want to prove it, it is a prerequisite that we rate therapists' treatment adherence and competence. There is no way around it. Accordingly, we are developing a manual and a mentalization-based group therapy adherence and competence scale, like the previous one for individual psychotherapy, in cooperation with Anthony Bateman and colleagues from Sweden and Denmark. Hopefully, this will be finished in 2012. It is an exciting piece of work. Group sessions have a laboratory flavour. Levels of mentalization can be operationalised and to what extent a group, and its therapists, do their job, is also open for measurement.

Research in group analysis has been hampered by too lose a definition as to what counts as good group analytic practice. A stricter definition of the structure and guiding therapeutic principles of group therapy for borderline patients might stimulate process research, which also may turn out to be relevant to the practice of group ana- lytic psychotherapy.

Taken together, imposing a certain structure, introducing privileged themes and advocating a certain therapeutic stance, implies a considerable deviance from commonly agreed upon group analytic principles. The underlying assumption is that group analytic psychotherapy is appropriate for better functioning patients, but that it is not a generic psychotherapy that works well for all type of patients. It must be structured differently when it comes to poorly functioning patients with specified pathologies. This means that what we are proposing here, is not a generic mentalization-based group treatment either. It is specifically designed for patients with prominent borderline features, while patients with hard-core avoidant PD might need another kind of group therapy.

When writing this memorial lecture, I have been concerned with what Foulkes might have said to the thoughts being outlined here. They may sound a bit heretic. However, our colleague Dieter Nitzgen has alerted me to a paragraph in the first textbook of Foulkes:

> By following the group, I do not mean I fall in with everything the group wants. If the group's tendency is towards the solution of its problems, I follow it. If it is away from that solution, I counteract this tendency by counter-arrangements. (Foulkes, 1948: 27)

A benign comment would be that we are engaged in systemizing some counter-arrangements, specifically designed for a certain kind of pathology. It is important that these developments occur in dialogue with group analysis. Group analytic theory and practice are always in our minds when we discuss, try out new kind of interventions and study the video recordings of our small-scale experiments. We are acutely aware that we are not just adding some new kind of interventions. These interventions and the theory behind them affect the group matrix as such and we need group analytic theory to reflect upon and understand the dynamic implications.

References

Baldwin, S. A., Wampold, B. E. & Imel, Z. E. (2007). Untangling the alliance- outcome correlation: Exploring the relative importance of therapist and patient variability in the alliance. *Journal of Consulting and Clinical Psychology,* 75(6): 842–852.

Bateman, A. & Fonagy, P. (1999). Effectiveness of partial hospitalization in the treatment of borderline personality disorder: A randomized controlled trial. *American Journal of Psychiatry*, 156(10): 1563–1569.

Bateman, A. & Fonagy, P. (2001). Treatment of borderline personality disorder with psychoanalytically oriented partial hospitalization: An 18-month follow- up. *American Journal of Psychiatry,* 158(1): 36–42.

Bateman, A. & Fonagy, P. (2006). *Mentalization-based Treatment for Borderline Personality Disorder. A Practical Guide.* Oxford: Oxford University Press.

Bateman, A. & Fonagy, P. (2009). Randomized controlled trial of outpatient mentalization-based treatment versus structured clinical management for borderline personality disorder. *American Journal of Psychiatry,* 166(12): 1355–1364.

Bateman, A. W. & Fonagy, P. (2004). *Psychotherapy for Borderline Personality Disorder. Mentalization-based Treatment.* Oxford: Oxford University Press.

Bogdan, R. J. (2000). *Minding Minds: Evolving a Reflexive Mind by Interpreting Others.* Cambridge: The MIT Press.

Corballis, M. C. (2007). The evolution of language: From hand to mouth. In M. S. Platek, J. P. Keenan & T. K. Shackelford (Eds.), *Evolutionary Cognitive Neuroscience*. Cambridge: The MIT Press.

Fonagy, P., Gergely, G., Jurist, E. L. & Target, M. (2003). *Affect Regulation, Mentalization, and the Development of the Self.* New York: Other Press.

Fonagy, P. & Luyten, P. (2009). A developmental, mentalization-based approach to the understanding and treatment of borderline personality disorder. *Developmental Psychopathology,* 21(4): 1355–1381.

Foulkes, S. H. (1948). *Introduction to Group-Analytic Psychotherapy*. London: Heinemann Medical Books.

Foulkes, S. H. (1973). The group as matrix of the individual's mental life. In L. R.Wolberg & E. K. Schwartz (Eds.), *Group Therapy 1973*. New York: Intercontinental Medical Book Corporation.

Foulkes, S. H. & Anthony, E. J. (1957). *Group Psychotherapy: The Psycho-analytic Approach*. Oxford and England: Penguin Books.

Giesen-Bloo, J., van Dyck, R., Spinhoven, P., van Tilburg, W., Dirksen, C., van Asselt, T. et al. (2006). Outpatient psychotherapy for borderline personality disorder. Randomized trial of schema-focused therapy versus transference-focused psychotherapy. *Archives of General Psychiatry,* 63(6): 649–658.

Gullestad, F., Wilberg, T., Klungsøyr, O., Urnes, Ø. & Karterud, S. (2012). Is treatment in a day hospital step-down program superior to outpatient individual psychotherapy for patients with personality disorders? – Results from a randomized clinical trial comparing different modalities. *Psychotherapy Research,* 22(4), 426–441.

Gullestad, F. S., Johansen, M. S., Høglend, P., Karterud, S. & Wilberg, T. (2013). Mentalization as a moderator of treatment effects: Findings from a randomized clinical trial for personality disorders, *Psychotherapy Research,* 23(6): 674–689.

Heidegger, M. (1927). *Being and Time*. New York: Harper and Row, 1962.

Hummelen, B., Pedersen, G., Wilberg, T., Kvarstein, E. & Karterud, S. The outcome of group psychotherapy for personality disorders. Are there differences between groups? unpublished article.

Hummelen, B., Wilberg, T. & Karterud, S. (2007). Interviews of female patients with borderline personality disorder who dropped out of group psychotherapy. *International Journal of Group Psychotherapy,* 57(1): 67–91.

Iacobini, M. & Mazziotta, J. C. (2007). Mirror neuron system: Basic findings and clinical applications. *Annals of Neurology*, 62(3): 213–218.

Karterud, S. (1999). *Gruppeanalyse og psykodynamisk gruppepsykoterapi*. Oslo: Pax forlag.

Karterud, S. & Bateman, A. (2010). *Manual for Mentaliseringsbasert terapi (MBT) og MBT vurderingsskala. Versjon individualterapi*. Oslo: Gyldendal Akademisk.

Karterud, S., Pedersen, G., Bjordal, E., Brabrand, J., Friis, S., Haaseth, O., Haavald- sen, G., Irion, T., Leirvåg, H., Tørum, A. & Urnes, Ø. (2003). Day treatment of patients with personality disorders: Experiences from a Norwegian treatment research network. *Journal of Personality Disorders,* 17(3): 243–262.

Karterud, S., Pedersen, G., Johansen, M. S., Johansen, P., Schlüter, C., Engen, M., Wilberg, T., Urnes, Ø. & Bateman, A. (2013). The mentalization-based treatment adherence and competence scale (MBT-ACS): Development, structure and reliability. *Psychotherapy Research,* 23(6): 705–717.

Karterud, S., Wilberg, T. & Urnes, Ø. (2010). *Personlighetspsykiatri*. Oslo: Gyl-dendal Akademisk.

Karterud, S. W. (1998). The group, self, empathy, intersubjectivity and herme- neutics: A group analytic perspective. In I. Harwood & M. Pines (Eds.), *Self Experiences in Groups. Intersubjective and Self Psychological Pathways to Human Understanding* (pp 83–98). London: Jessica Kingsley Publishers.

King-Casas, B., Sharp, C., Lomax-Bream, L., Lohrenz, T., Fonagy, P. & Montague, P. R. (2008). The rupture and repair of cooperation in borderline personality disorder. *Science*, 321: 806–810.

Kvarstein, E. & Karterud, S. (2013). Large variation of severity and five year course of symptom distress among patients with personality disorders. *Personality and Mental Health*, 7(4): 265–276. DOI: 10.1002/pmh.1226

Leichsenring, F. & Rabung, S. (2008). Effectiveness of long-term psychodynamic psycho-therapy: A meta-analysis. *JAMA*, 300(13): 1551–1565.

Lorentzen, S., Bøgwald, K. P. & Høglend, P. (2002). Change during and after long-term ana-lytic group psychotherapy. *International Journal of Group Psychotherapy*, 52: 419–429.

Nitsun, M. (2005). Destructive forces in group therapy. In L. Motherwell & J. Shay (Eds.), *Complex Dilemmas in Group Therapy* (pp. 115–125). New York: Brunner- Routledge.

Panksepp, J. (1998). *Affective Neuroscience: The Foundations of Human and Animal Emotions*. New York: Oxford University Press.

Perry, J. C., Banon, E. & Ianni, F. (1999). Effectiveness of psychotherapy for personality disorders. *American Journal of Psychiatry*, 156(9): 1312–1321.

Ricoeur, P. (1992). *Oneself as Another*. Chicago: The University of Chicago Press.

Roth, B. E., Stone, W. N. & Kibel, H. D. (1990). *The Difficult Patient in Group*. Madison: International Universities Press.

Siever, L. J. & Weinstein, L. N. (2009). The neurobiology of personality disorders: Implications for psychoanalysis. *Journal of the American Psychoanalytic Association*, 57: 361–398.

Zuroff, D. C., Kelly, A. C., Leybman, M. J., Blatt, S. J. & Wampold, B. E. (2010). Between-therapist and within-therapist differences in the quality of the Thera therapeutic rela-tionship: Effects on maladjustment and self-critical perfectionism. *Journal of Clinical Psychology*, 66(7): 681–697.

Chapter 5

A qualitative study of a mentalization-based group for borderline patients

Tryggve Inderhaug and Sigmund Karterud

Abstract

In this article we present a video-based explorative study of three consecutive Mentalization-based group therapy (MBT-G) sessions at a Norwegian Mental Health Centre. The aim of the study was to gain more knowledge about what kind of problems therapists would encounter when conducting MBT groups in an ordinary MHC, as part of the general public mental health services, without any connection to academic or university settings. MBT-G has its roots in group analytic psychotherapy but is modified to avoid the chaotic and destructive processes often encountered in groups consisting of severely personality disordered patients. Among the most notable differences from the Foulkesian group analytic approach are the therapists handling of authority and a "not-knowing stance" (as opposed to an interpretative stance). Contrary to our expectations we found the typical chaotic borderline group processes that MBT-G was designed to avoid. An in-depth examination of the data, employing qualitative Thematic Analysis, revealed that the therapists failed to establish themselves as authoritative leaders of the group and misconstrued the "not-knowing stance". We present transcripts of some typical sequences and discuss their clinical and therapeutic implications.

Material

The object for the study was a slow-open group that met 1.5 hours every week at a Mental Health Centre in Norway, as part of an established MBT programme. The choice of this particular group was based on convenience; it was part of the only MBT programme that existed close to the university site of the first author. As such, we do not claim it to be representative for MBT groups in general.

The group consisted of six female patients (age range 21–46) with borderline-type problems (being assessed by SCID-II). Thus, all patients had problems associated with emotion regulation, interpersonal relations and unstable sense of self. All had severely compromised social functioning, e.g., being unable to work or study. Four of the patients had been members of the group from the start, while the last

DOI: 10.4324/9781003625810-5

two had attended the group for ten and four sessions prior to data collection. All patients had supplementary individual therapy.

The group was conducted by two male therapists of psychodynamic orientation. One had been trained in group analysis for three years, supplemented with a two-year course in MBT-G. The other had followed a one-year course in MBT-G. The group therapists met with the individual therapists at team meetings every second week. The treatment team received external expert supervision about four times a year.

The researchers had no direct contact with the group and knew none of the patients in advance. The therapists informed the group about the research project, and patients read and signed an informed consent form before participating in the study. The therapists had previously video-recorded their sessions for supervisory purposes, so the research project did not represent deviation from existing routines. The research was approved by the Regional health research ethical committee.

Methods

While designing the study we decided to go beyond the question of whether the therapists adhered to the MBT manual or not (Karterud, 2012). We wanted to be open for hitherto unknown phenomena and, therefore advanced no propositions as to what we might find. We based our employment of Thematic Analysis (TA) on the accounts of Howitt and Cramer (2007) and Braun and Clarke (2006).

TA is basically a method for pattern finding. Themes derived from a TA organise and describe data. As a consequence of our theoretical framing, this study called for a detailed analysis of some aspects of the data (i.e. therapists interventions based on MBT principles), at expense of a rich description of the data as a whole.

Three subsequent therapy sessions, summing up to 4.5 hours of video data, were transcribed verbatim into about 59.000 words. All patients were given fictional names, and all content that could compromise their anonymity were altered.

As familiarization with data is vitally important in TA, the first author transcribed the data himself. The analysing process moved through transcription, repeated read-throughs of the transcripts, several meetings and discussions with supervisors, a feedback session with the therapists of the group in question, and ultimately ended while the first draft of the report was written (Inderhaug, 2013).

A limited number of themes which adequately reflected the textual data were identified through an analytic process of coding and integration of codes into themes. In the coding phase, the data was read over and over again, coding small segments with intuitive verbal descriptors. The codes were modified from one reading to the next, in the light of the developing apprehension of the totality of the data. In turn, themes that integrated substantial sets of the codes were formulated, and at last, the themes were compared to the items of the MBT-G Adherence and Competence scale (Karterud, 2012). The analytic process progressed from a descriptive phase, where the data was organised to show patterns without considering theoretical concerns, to an interpretative phase, where MBT theory served as an organizing principle for formulation of themes. In writing the present paper, we shortened and sharpened the results by conflating some of the themes presented in the initial report (Inderhaug, 2013).

The authors held a meeting with the therapists after having landed on some core themes in the analysis. When we had provided them with our feedback, the meeting took the form of a reflective dialogue where the therapists could help us adjust, develop, or confirm our understanding of the data.

Results

It was early apparent that the therapists met substantial challenges in dealing with this group. Borderline pathology suffused the discourse and the group processes, evident both in what patients talked about their life outside therapy and in the way they acted in the group. The content of the stories was often highly disturbing, describing chaotic family lives, substance abuse, violence, sexual transgressions and destructive acting out. The main therapeutic challenge appeared to be taking the reins in a group bordering on chaos. However, the therapists did not stand out as authoritative leaders. Instead, some patients had taken central positions in the group and dominated the discourse and the process.

The following four themes from the Thematic Analysis addressed the bulk of the therapists' challenges: (1) structuring the process, (2) interruptions/getting a word in, (3) determining importance, and (4) promoting pseudomentalization. Comparing these challenges to the MBT-G adherence and competence scale, we found that they related conceptually to two MBT-G principles. Theme 1 and 2 could be related to *managing authority,* and theme 3 and 4 to *exploration, curiosity* and *not-knowing stance*. The therapists seemed to have downplayed their role as experts on psychotherapy and group dynamics. On a phenomenological level, the tendencies of the therapists abdicating from the leadership and holding a mere supporting role in the group could be associated with the not-knowing stance in MBT. In the following we will elucidate the themes and related principles, starting with managing authority.

Before text examples are presented, it should be mentioned that one of the therapists (T1) is a recurrent character in the chosen transactions. T1 was more involved in relevant transactions, while the other (T2) adhered less to MBT principles. Furthermore, a few patients were clearly dominant, both in terms of shaping the group dynamics and in mere verbal activity. The tendencies we want to highlight here stands out most clearly in the transactions involving these patients, and necessarily, they are overrepresented in the text examples. As space limitations do not allow us to present longer transactions, we jump straight into complex and at times chaotic transactions. The reader may find it difficult to grasp what the group is talking about. In fact, we were tempted to correct the transcript in order to make it more comprehensible for the reader. However, that would distort the discourse as it actually took place. The discourse *was* often chaotic and difficult to understand. Still, the main points we want to make concerns the process more than the content of the transactions, and we believe the relevant processes are well illustrated in the text examples.

Managing authority

In MBT-G, the therapists should take a firm stance by expressing in simple words the tasks and goals of the group (e.g., what are expected from the group members, why the therapists will work in certain manners, etc.). The challenges associated with managing authority in this group will be presented through the following themes: 1) *structuring the process,* and 2) *interruptions/getting a word in.*

Structuring the process: Each session should optimally start with "minding the group" and "building bridges" to the previous group session. It is a strategy that aims to compensate for the lack of self-structure among the members and to promote a better group cohesion. It reminds the members of what happened, emphasizing that the recapitulation is a result of the therapists minding endeavour ("this is what we have thought since last time"), and conveys what the therapists have found important to mention. Next, the therapists should ask for initiatives, preferably difficult interpersonal events to be explored in the group. The next structuring challenge for the therapists is terminating the work around one patient and opening up for another protagonist. Finally, the therapists should terminate the session in an organised way. In the following, we provide examples from the opening phase, the mid phase and the end of the group.

In this group the therapists omitted the feedback from the last meeting. They went straight on to organise themes and events. The patients had obvious problems with this phase. They took long to recall their events, and if they did, they usually were not able to keep it brief and started to give detailed accounts as if the therapeutic work had already started. The therapist's struggled hard to organise this phase, as illustrated by this sequence from about eight minutes into a session. Sarah is presenting a theme that she may want to work with in the group and the therapists are trying to reach a conclusion in order to move on in the planning of the session:

Sarah:	and dating is like, so stiff! Getting home to take a shower, dress up, and fair enough I like that, I do, but-
T1:	but wait a minute, wait, Sarah, wait! Sarah! Sarah, wait a minute …
Sarah:	it's so, it's so stiff! (laughs)
T1:	hold on Sarah! (smiles) ee …
	(scattered laughter)
Sarah:	but is it important?
T1:	is-is, shall we- is – is your relation to him an important subject to you, and how it has been?
Sarah:	no, we don't have a relation yet
T1:	no okay, but okay, it's eh, I'm not speaking of a relation as a romantic relationship, but considering, you have a relation to him because you've

met him, and it means something to you. And it is a relation in that respect, is what I meant. Becau- That is, not a relation as in a romantic relation, but your relation, considering that he, is a man who arouse some feelings

Sarah: oh yes, but I fear that I will end up with the same thing I had with Chris, because, I already get a sense that …

T1: yes, yes (gestures: wait, stop, enough already)

T2: this sounds like an important event

Sarah: it seems to be one of those warning signs, with all this, like fixation on appearance

T1: yes, but hey, but wait a minute

Sarah: yeah! I'm waiting!

Isabel: (laughs)

T1: yes (laughs)

Isabel: there's no way to stop you, when you've started!

Sarah: (laughs loudly, puts her hand in front of her face) aah! I feel like I'm … (unintelligible)

T1: but perhaps, eh like, perhaps it's important for you to have a look on this matter?

Isabel: it would be even more abnormal if you did not feel like this! If not you would have gone blindly into something with someone, one that you might as well had found completely uninteresting, just to see if there was anything to it

Sarah: yes, but I'm thinking it's better …

T1: hold on! Okey! (gestures: stop, wait)

T2: now we're working!

T1: now we're working again, let us –s-s-say this is a theme

T2: yes, it sounds very interesting

T1: are there anyone else who have eh … anything?

The length of the opening phases varies considerably among groups. In well organised groups it is fairly rapid, and patients and therapists come to some kind of agreement within five-ten minutes. Ten minutes after the sequence above, the group had not yet started working, bearing witness of problems with the alliance and agreement on the basic group principles.

In the next sequence the therapists are terminating a turn with a designated patient. T1 has been trying to stop Sarah for about four minutes in order to move on to a new patient. Sarah is clearly mocking him, and she is fully aware that she has been ignoring him for some time.

T1: I'm thinking we might be stopping there

Sarah: yes, we've stopped several times! (smiles and imitates T1's «stopping-gesture») «we'll stop here!» «we'll stop here!»

	(unintelligible comments and laughter)
Sarah:	no, I'll zip my mouth now (straightens herself up in the chair)
T1:	you get eager, Sarah
Sarah:	yeeah, but-eh …
Isabel:	but that's a good thing!-
Sarah:	but you'll have to praise me, I've been good and worked out a great deal
T1:	yees (hesitant)
Isabel:	I think you're doing great
Sarah:	and I've been working on loads of other stuff in the group too
Isabel:	I get really impressed with you, when you're doing well in your job, and you've been working out and have regular activities and stuff!
Sarah:	yes
Isabel:	it's got to be just wonderful!
Sarah:	yes…
Isabel:	(laughs)
Sarah:	but then I feel sorry for myself some times
T2:	(laughs)
Isabel:	who doesn't?
T1:	yeah, okay! Shall we move on?
T2:	(laughs)
Isabel:	not to render it commonplace though
Sarah:	no, I know! I know, I get what you're saying, everybody feels the same. I'm normal! (looks at T2)
T2:	mhm (nods)
Sarah:	I'm one among many (smiles) I'm not …
Isabel:	(laughs loudly)
Sarah:	I'm not on my spaceship anymore!
T2:	(laughs)
Rose:	(laughs)
T1:	(smiles) I'm getting the feeling that eh, I've been repeating myself a number of times now
Isabel:	(laughs on)
Sarah:	okay, zip! ("zips" her mouth)
T1:	where were we?

The following sequence is from the end of a session. Rose is stopped in the middle of a frantic effort to pack in more details about her life in the very last minute. The result is that the group is ended abruptly, not leaving room for a summary from the therapists.

T1:	*(draws his breath) okey*
Rose:	*yes, cause now we're … bhjgc*

T1:	*it's – it's …*
Rose:	*we're watching some detective series on TV, right? And Kirsten comes in halfway through, because her girl wouldn't sleep. She had to lay down with her and sing, until she fell asleep! (frowns)*
T1:	*clock is ticking*
Rose:	*where the hell is normality then?*
T1:	*well, so you say. Clock is ticking. And we could be looking at many things here, cause I can hear that ...*
Rose:	*could sit for one more hour!*
T1:	*sounds as if, there is a lot being stirred up here, and it gives rise to many episodes that have provoked you. Eeeh, and I think it's great that you bring it up… Think it's …*
Rose:	*-it's just whining*
T1:	*is it just whining?*
Rose:	*so now it's all about doing a turnaround, now, to begin thinking about myself again. And that's, something I have been thinking of a lot, that's something I find so hard now. Because that's the way I am, now I'm all grumpy and irritable, and to make matters worse, daddy just fell, because he was moving last Saturday. (Looks at her wrist-watch) I'll hurry up!*
T1:	*(laughs)*
Rose:	*He fractured his kneecap! And boy do I feel bad for not visiting my mum in the Easter holydays, because we had visitors at home the whole time. So now I have, Thomas is calling me constantly, and Jesus I'm driven crazy! So I think I have to go off to somewhere. Go to Hawaii or someplace like that*
Trudy:	*Spain …*
Rose:	*be gone for a month. Or two, or three, or four.*
Sarah:	*and why not?*
T2:	*(laughing) take off or take a stand*
T1:	*okey! That's it for today.*

Structuring the process provides ample opportunities for stimulating metacognition, e.g., by not focusing on the content, but on structural principles that are decisive for the very process of dialogue and mentalizing in a group (e.g., "were we able to tune in on this story?"). By discussing these principles, the members ideally may come to internalise and own them, and thus, this part of the discourse may contribute to the alliance. In this group, the therapists did not stimulate (or had they given up?) this kind of higher order reflection.

Interruptions/getting a word in: There was a high rate of interruptions on the part of the patients, and the therapists often had troubles getting a word in. In advance of the following sequence, T1 had made many unsuccessful attempts to slow down the ongoing interaction. He opens with excusing himself for interrupting Sarah but ends up being ignored and not getting his point through.

T1:	*I wond … I'm wondering, I think I interrupted you earlier, Sarah, eh … if that's the case I'm sorry*
Sarah:	*(shakes her head)*
Isabel:	*(to Rose, while T1 speaks) not to be nasty*
Rose:	*no! But I see what you're saying*
Sarah:	*(to T1) what?*
T1:	*I thought … uh, you said something like «what can youth understand? »*
Sara:	*yes*
T1:	*(draws his breath) wha, how …*
Sarah:	*I think she may have too high expectations of them*
Rose:	*now I tell you what, I don't think so! That's the least you can expect from someone who's turned twenty years old!*
Sarah:	*nooo …*
Rose:	*but – but youth, they are all different too!*
T1:	*yes, wha …*
Rose:	*that's, they are*
Sarah:	*you must bear in mind that people express love differently!*
Rose:	*yeah!*
Sarah:	*like Jesus, you can't, like I understand that you may have …*
Rose:	*but! Yes that's exact … that's exactly what they …*
Sarah:	*what kinda expectations, if you have expectations it's just the same as being let down*
T1:	*but wha …*
Sarah:	*you're better off having no expectations and let them show you love in their own way!*
Rose:	*and that's what I think I'm doing too, cause that's how I am, and that has nothing to do with the kids, and it can be something that, maybe something is supposed to take place and I think «no, it's not gonna happen anyway»*
T1:	*(draws his breath)*
Isabel:	*that's something to remind them of too then. What you actually do for them! Because they're … most kids are certainly, spoiled!*
Sarah:	*yes but how are they supposed to know, and we acknow… or express love when you don't tell them what you want then?! It's like you have …*
Rose:	*I have told them!*
Sarah:	*yes but, once then!*
Rose:	*no, I have told them several times after that too*
T1:	*(says something that drowns in Rose's speech)*

(In the sequel: T1 does not get a word in)

Not-knowing stance

We will present two aspects of the therapists' challenges associated with the not-knowing stance. These challenges are: 1) *determining importance*, and 2) therapists' unwittingly *promoting pseudomentalization* by stimulating patients to mentalize on the basis of chaotic narratives replete with multiple problems.

Determining importance: The therapists conducted the group by spending a long time (20-30 minutes) on the opening phase of each session. Partly, this could be understood as a consequence of the therapists not holding an expert position in the group, because a major challenge was confusion among the patients about which topic to present. Before the following segment, Sarah has just been narrating about her emerging relationship with a new man. We understand from what she was telling earlier in the session that relationships are problematic to her in many ways, but as T1 asks her what she is afraid will happen, she answers that she is afraid to get stomach trouble and be embarrassed. T1 draws on what Sarah said earlier when he asserts that there is another, perhaps more important aspect to the situation.

Sarah: *and I'm thinking like (smiles)…*
T1: *but-eh is that what you are most anxious about now, because …*
Sarah: *I'm mostly …*
T1: *I-eh was a little surprised with your answer, cause you you …*
T2: *m-m-*
T1: *I would have thought you'd say «I'm afraid that …*
Sarah: *not s …*
T1: *-I'll engage in a relationship that eh, is not making me feel, not making me feel good, and that is not good for me, and that may lead to me starting drinking again». That's what I would have thought was your answer*
Sarah: *no, that's no problem*
T1: *you're not afraid of that?*
Sarah: *no like, I'm such a badass when it comes to that stuff, I … I'll just 'pyssh' (gestures «tossing something over her shoulder») «enough of that», but-eh …*
T1: *what do you think about that I thoug-e-about my understanding of the situation?*
Sarah: *I understand that, because that's what's normal, but I feel that by now I've been working so hard with myself. I'm that independent, that I have … I'm standing on my own two feet, dammit. I used to be terribly emotionally dependent on Chris, but no more of that. I refuse to be emotionally dependent on another human being, or to be dependent on another human being in any way. Eeeem … and I have so many other things in my life that I've filled my life with, so there is no, even if I like meet him a couple of times more and find it's not working out, I'm thinking «well well, but at least it's one more lesson learned», like it's …*

T1:	*what are you others thinking about this?*
Sarah:	*like it's not, life's not over*
T2:	*no*
T1:	*what are you thinking?*
Rose:	*well, it sounds like terrific and you seem so incredibly strong*
T2:	*-how can you figure out how much he is drinking then?*

We see that T1 is cautiously questioning Sarah's focus on physical and somatic aspects of the situation. Instead of being more persistent, he calls on the group for support. T1 is clearly on to something, he *knows* that there are important mental aspects to this. He hints towards alternative perspectives but is also hesitant and "not-knowing". He asks the group what they are thinking; apparently hoping they will pick up on his cue. Unfortunately, the other patients (or T2) seldom follow him, and he ends up not getting his point through.

Promoting pseudomentalization: One of the most frequent interventions from T1 was, on the basis of patient narratives, to ask the group what they were thinking about the situation being described, what they believed was going on in the minds of the subjects of the narrative, what they were feeling, and why they may have been behaving the way they were. From a mentalizing point of view, these are perfectly legitimate questions. However, as a consequence of poorly structured processes, the information the patients were asked to use as a basis for mentalization was often extremely vague. Upon T1's questions, this vagueness led patients to make general assumptions, suggest stereotypical explanations of what was going on, and often simply suggest solutions to the problems they were presented with. What seemed to be efforts to mentalize were often not grounded in an appreciation of real events, but rather on phantasies and loose assumptions. In other words, the patients' mentalization was often not based on the results of conjoint explorations of subjective realities and appeared therefore more like pseudomentalization.

The sequences we have already quoted contain several examples of pseudomentalization. In the following example, Trudy has just finished a complex story (observe T1's first response) which becomes interpreted by clichés. The behaviour is believed to be a consequence of unresolved grief/sorrow without any evidence of it.

T1:	*(expires:) hoi!*
T2:	*m-m*
Trudy:	*but not that exact episode though, the condom-stuff, because then ... I had already caught him cheating, so it was already over, but I had the key to his apartment, so that was no sweat. And eventually she got fired*
T1:	*but... there- there's been terribly much going on here*
Trudy:	*m-m, (laughs a little) there's usually some action*
T1:	*a-a-and, what are you (the group) thinking? Eeeh ... How do you think Trudy has been doing?*

(Trudy laughs)
Rose: *you do have a fierce temper*
Trudy: *yes I do*
Sarah: *it's because you're not able to free yourselves from the sorrow, I think. So you get angry instead. There's always something lying under the anger*
Trudy: *-but I've always had my temp …*
Sarah: *-There's always something lying under the anger!!*

Calling on the group to mentalize is a technique that underscores the principle of therapist-patient equality. The therapists are often not in a better position than the patients to make sense of mental states. However, the therapists are often in a better position to know *what information is needed* to properly grasp what is going on. The preparation of the scene, so to speak, is an important task in MBT-G. Therapists should assist group members in clarifying relevant scenes, and then stimulate curiosity about what went on in the minds of the involved people. Our impression in this group was often that if the therapists themselves were to make any sense out of the "hotchpotch" presented in many of the sequences, their mentalization would be just as much guesswork, that is, pseudomentalization.

Discussion

In this study of a MBT group at a MHC, we found chaotic group processes of types that are well known from the literature (Pines, 1990; Marziali & Munroe-Blum, 1994; Hummelen, Wilberg & Karterud, 2007). The group was conducted by two therapists who had previous training in group analysis and MBT. We could observe that one of them (T1) consistently tried to apply MBT principles. However, the effect upon the group seemed minimal with respect to constructing scenarios that were useful for conjoint exploration and mentalizing.

We found that several themes from the Thematic Analysis were related to two principles in the MBT-G manual: managing authority and the not-knowing stance. The therapists struggled to manage their authority in an efficient fashion, and also exhibited what we conceived as an exaggerated not-knowing attitude. That is, the therapists were seen to adhere little to the item "managing authority", while the "not-knowing stance" was overplayed. The therapists seemed to be trapped between two models. With one leg in each camp, they did not practice group analytic psychotherapy, nor did they practice MBT-G.

The findings of this study illustrate some difficulties therapists encounter when trying to establish themselves as leaders of a certain communicational structure. We observed how the therapists were overheard, not paid attention to, interrupted, and at times ridiculed. As outlined in the companion paper (Karterud, 2015), this is a form of discourse where no development of social cognition can take place. Some patients had become very influential in shaping this discourse and the therapists' feared aggressive outbursts if they were to challenge it. Consequently, trapped in a lack of therapeutic alliance, they became reticent about their endeavour to transform the therapeutic process to conform to MBT-G standards.

We suggest that some of the difficulties that the therapists encountered can be explained by competing theoretical models in their minds, being embodied and acted out through a more mentalization-based approach by T1 and a more psychodynamic approach by T2. We still contend that group analysis and MBT-G are not contradictory models of group psychotherapy (Karterud, 2011). We have witnessed several fruitful hybrids. A working hypothesis is that the better mental functioning the group members exhibit, the more appropriate are group analytic principles, while increasing mentalizing difficulties call for MBT techniques.

The study concerns three meetings in a MCH MBT group, and the findings may not be valid for this group over time. We may have observed a stressful period in the life of the group. We should neither generalise the finding to other MCH MBT groups. Nevertheless, we recognise a theoretical and therapeutic tension here that may have relevance for many groups. Therefore, we have taken the opportunity to exploit these group experiences for the purpose of clarifying crucial theoretical and practical issues. Through this study, we have also become more alert to sources of confusion on the themes of authority and structure versus the not-knowing stance, and it has helped us to clarify issues that earn more consideration in MBT-G training, and possibly in group analytic training as well.

References

Braun, V. & Clarke, V. (2006). Using thematic analysis in psychology. *Qualitative Research in Psychology*, 3(2): 77–101.

Howitt, D. & Cramer, D. (2007). *Introduction to Research Methods in Psychology*. 2nd revised edition. New York: Pearson Education.

Hummelen, B., Wilberg, T. & Karterud, S. (2007). Interviews of female patients with borderline personality disorder who dropped out of group psychotherapy. *International Journal of Group Psychotherapy*, 57(1): 67–91.

Inderhaug, T. S. (2013). *Challenges in Mentalization–based Group Therapy (MBT-G): A Video-based Explorative Case Study*. (Graduate thesis). Trondheim: The Norwegian University of Science and Technology.

Karterud, S. (2011). Constructing and mentalizing the matrix. *Group Analysis*, 44(4): 1–17

Karterud, S. (2012). *Manual for mentaliseringbasert gruppeterapi (MBT-G)*. Oslo: Gyldendal Akademisk.

Karterud, S. (2015). On structure and leadership in MBT-G and group analysis. *Group Analysis*, 48(2): 137–149.

Marsiali, E. & Munroe-Blum, H. (1994). *Interpersonal Group Psychotherapy for Borderline Personality Disorder*. New York: Basic Books.

Pines, M. (1990). *Group Analytic Psychotherapy and the Borderline Patient*. In B. E. Roth, W. N. Stone, & H. D. Kibel (Eds.), *The Difficult Patient in Group*. Madison: International Universities Press.

Chapter 6

On structure and leadership in MBT-G and group analysis

Sigmund Karterud

Abstract

Mentalization-based group therapy (MBT-G) has its roots in group analytic psychotherapy. In this article, modifications are described that might suit the needs of more disturbed personality disordered patients and counteract the chaotic and destructive processes often encountered in groups dominated by these patients. The MBT-G principles of leadership, structure and authority are discussed in comparison with group analysis. Clinical and research evidence indicate that prerequisites for sound social cognition are likely to become violated when efforts of communicational re-education take place in a group composed of personality disordered individuals who have received minimal instructions on how to proceed. Such experiments likely end up in disconnected speech and utterances, aborted stories conveying fragments of experiences, emotional outbursts and activation of psychic equivalence, malign projective identifications, sequences of pseudo-mentalization, experiences of not being heard and respected, as well hopelessness and disillusionment. Such situations call for therapists, not as conductors, but as competent leaders who model a kind of parental-like authority. This parental-like authority is less concerned with what is right or wrong, as how to reach truth about oneself and others. Philosophically, such an attitude is grounded in communicational ethics (e.g., P. Grice and J. Habermas) which concerns the implicit ethos of communication between humans, e.g., a wish for communication and conveying honest messages, a concern for truth, a respect for the dialog partner, active listening and an effort to understand the partner's mental state and point of view, etc. This kind of communication does not come by nature. It is hard won achievements of cultural (group) evolution. The concept of mentalizing stance belongs to this tradition of ideas. Basically, the idea is that by the individual group members striving to become a member of the mentalizing group self, i.e. the work group aspect of the group, one must develop one's social cognition. Or phrased in another way: the development of social cognition (narration, attention, focusing, inhibitory control, affect consciousness, metacognition, mentalizing, integration, etc.) is likely to be a result of one's efforts to become a member of the group self. This logic is supported by modern theories of evolution of thinking, self-consciousness and culture.

DOI: 10.4324/9781003625810-6

Mentalization-based treatment (MBT), originally designed for the treatment of borderline personality disorder (BPD), has proved efficient in randomised controlled trials and naturalistic studies (Bateman & Fonagy, 2001, 2009; Bales et al., 2012; Rossouw & Fonagy, 2012; Kvarstein et al., 2014). MBT is a conjoint treatment, combining individual (MBT-I) and group therapy (MBT-G). Recently, manuals for MBT-I (Karterud & Bateman, 2010), MBT pscyhoeducative group therapy (Karterud & Bateman, 2011), and MBT-G (Karterud, 2012) have been published in Norwegian. These treatment manuals follow the recommended standards of Luborsky and Barber (1993), by including theoretical background, treatment principles, therapeutic techniques with specific examples, in addition to rating scales for therapist adherence and competence.

The main objective of MBT is to enhance patients' inherent capacity for mentalizing for the purpose of improving their intersubjective competence, and thereby enhancing their sense of self cohesion and identity (Fonagy et al., 2011). MBT requires the cultivation of a mentalizing stance in both therapist and patients, which entails a humble acknowledgement of not-knowing, patience in identifying different perspectives, as well as an active effort to make detailed accounts of experiences rather than explaining them (Bateman & Fonagy, 2004). The patients are ideally engaged in a mentalizing discourse where beliefs, feelings and interpersonal transactions are challenged to bring about changes in perspective, while solutions and answers play subordinate roles (Karterud & Bateman, 2010).

There is a large literature and a rich clinical tradition on treatment of borderline patients by group psychotherapy (Roth, Stone & Kibel, 1990). Such treatment is considered difficult and demands competent therapists and well-functioning groups (Marziali & Munroe-Blum, 1994). Typical clinical issues are how to deal with splitting and malign projective identification, and in particular how to avoid that these phenomena infect the group as a whole (Pines, 1990). The textbook literature clearly advices therapists to compose their groups in a balanced way, by not adding more than a few borderline patients (Rutan, Stone & Shay, 2007; Yalom & Leszcz, 2005).

The group psychotherapy landscape has been changed recent years by public mental health services imposing group therapists to accept poorly functioning patients, thereby forcing them to abandon previous politics of selecting patients according to established principles of suitability. We are more often than before witnessing groups where many of the members suffer severe personality disorders (Karterud & Wilberg, 2007).

The response to this situation has been a development of treatment techniques that might counteract the problems created when all the members of a group have serious problems of self-cohesion and interpersonal functioning. A common strategy has been to abolish the principle of free group association and providing more structure to the group processes. For example, the group component of dialectical behavioural therapy (DBT) is very structured and defined as a device for developing social skills (Linehan, 1993). The "Group schema therapy for borderline personality disorder" is also a highly structured cognitive oriented group therapy, where the agenda is defined by the therapists according to a predefined sequence of goals (Farrell & Shaw, 2012). However, MBT-G, which evolved through modifications of group analysis, still adhere to the principle of group *psychotherapy through the group process* (Karterud, 2011).

Both in the theoretical and empirical literature on MBT, the individual component of the treatment is well covered, while the group component has received comparatively less attention (Karterud & Bateman, 2011). Unfortunately, the recent and comprehensive manual by Karterud (2012) is only available in Norwegian. In this manual, general principles of MBT-G are formulated with an emphasis on the significance of the mentalizing stance in groups. It also includes detailed descriptions of 19 specified treatment principles, which constitute the core of a MBT-G adherence and competence rating scale. Ten of these principles are similar to items in the manual for individual MBT (Karterud et al., 2013): 1) Engagement, interest and warmth; 2) Exploration, curiosity and not-knowing stance; 3) Challenging unwarranted beliefs; 4) Regulating arousal; 5) Acknowledging good mentalization; 6) Dealing with pretend mode; 7) Dealing with psychic equivalence; 8) Keeping an affect focus; 9) practicing "stop and rewind", and 10) Focus on the relation between the therapists and the group members ("transference").

In addition, there are 9 group specific items. These items address specific structural elements which are of vital importance for the group as a whole:

1) Managing the boundaries of the group;
2) Regulating the phases of the group;
3) Initiating and fulfilling turn-taking;
4) Engaging the group members in mentalizing interpersonal events embedded in the narratives of the turn-taking;
5) Identifying and mentalizing events in the group;
6) Care for the group and each member;
7) Managing authority;
8) Stimulating and assisting the group in discussions on themes relevant for the group culture;
9) Cooperation with the co-therapist.

The purpose of these principles is to provide the therapists with tools that will make it possible to conduct a dynamic group even with poorly functioning patients. MBT-G structuring principles can be understood as a response to the inherent dangers of chaos and destructivity associated with including many borderline patients in groups. MBT-G has its roots in group analysis and psychodynamic group psychotherapy. These group therapies all share a common therapeutic principle in that significant intersubjective transactions unfolding in the group are actively brought to attention and explored–a hallmark of dynamic therapy. However, MBT-G parts ways with other long-held dynamic principles. The most noteworthy deviation is that the therapists take responsibility for structuring each session, explicitly invite for exploration of interpersonal events, and make active efforts to regulate current emotional arousal. Furthermore, the roles and tasks of the patients and the therapists, the objective of the group and the way to reach this objective, are more clearly defined and explicated for patients in MBT-G.

A session typically starts out with a short recapitulation of the previous session ("building bridges" and "minding the group"). Then, for the sake of structuring the present session, patients are asked to signal their need for time and space in the group, typically centred on significant (interpersonal) events from the last week. Thus, MBT-G encourages *turn-taking* as a central therapeutic and organizing principle, which puts it in contrast to the typical unstructured psychodynamic group therapy. It is important to underline that this turn-taking is not equal to "individual therapy in groups". It is still dynamic group psychotherapy, however focused in turns on designated patients and their intersubjective and emotional problems. The manual contains detailed discussions on how to conduct such interpersonally focused turn-taking, without creating a dependency group in Bion' sense (Bion, 1961) or resorting to a kind of individual therapy with spectators (Karterud, 2012).

A typical MBT-G session will revolve around a constant effort to understand specific situations from the patients' life, or situations unfolding in the group here-and-now. Interpersonal events are probably more highly prioritised in MBT-G than in other psychodynamic group therapies. The therapists' chief task is to stimulate patients to mentalize these events, and further, to create and sustain a mentalizing discourse in the group. A mentalizing discourse is hallmarked by an emphasis on details of events that allows for constructive imagination and realisation of what goes on in the minds of the subjects. Thus, it is necessary to be specific about what happened, at what time, who was involved, what the involved persons were doing or saying, and what the narrator was thinking and feeling. The patients should learn to sketch interpersonal situations so that both therapists and the other patients are able to tune in on the transactions. For that purpose, it is advisable to dive into single events instead of sketching many events superficially.

By a skilful practice of the above-mentioned principles, the aim is to construe a *mentalizing group culture*. As patients in MBT-G conjointly meets with their individual therapists, the group therapists can intensify the interpersonal emphasis in the group sessions, leaving in-depth intrapersonal exploration and social support to the individual sessions. In principle, the group situation is an excellent arena for exploring interpersonal events and enhancing the capacity to mentalize. The challenging task for the therapists is to realise this potential. With a group consisting of persons with severe personality disorders, this is difficult.

Managing authority is a therapeutic principle specific to MBT-G, not being part of the individual treatment manual. The group manual discusses in length how the therapists' authority may be challenged by different aspects of borderline pathology, e.g., by devaluating or aggressive patients, and in general by powerful projective identifications. It is important for therapists to remember the fact that they have invited the patients to participate in a specifically designed project, with a particular purpose and a set of ground rules. The therapists should lead the group with a firm hand and make sure that issues of relevance for the therapeutic project are attended to. MBT-G is far from the group analytic ideals of "trust the group" and "leave it to the group". When patients derail the process, the therapist should interrupt the ongoing transaction and get the group back on track. In contrast to more typical psychodynamic group therapies, MBT group therapists should provide the group with structure and guidance and be more explicitly responsible for the therapeutic process.

One precaution that is given special attention in both individual and group MBT is that the therapist should not stand out as an omnipotent expert with a privileged knowledge of what is "really" going on in the group or in the mind of its members. Instead, the therapeutic stance should be curious, active, empathic, and at times challenging. The therapists should be focused on the patients' mind and their ongoing intersubjective transactions in an engaged, questioning, and not-knowing way (Bateman & Fonagy, 2006a). *The principle of not-knowing* is believed to stimulate the curiosity and engagement of the patients, and ultimately to foster mentalization. It is considered potentially anti-therapeutic to take on an expert attitude with respect to the content of the mind, as the patients may accept a therapist's point of view indiscriminately, following his lead while leaving their own feelings of what is important behind (Bateman & Fonagy, 2006b).

The manual of MBT-G was developed by this author in cooperation with Anthony Bateman and several skilled group analysts from prominent treatment units in the Nordic countries that had extensive experience with BPD patients (Karterud, 2012). The development was based upon extensive examinations of video-recordings of ongoing groups and experiments with different techniques and treatment principles, in particular groups from the Department of Personality Psychiatry, Oslo University Hospital. The manual was revised several times before reaching an acceptable consensus. MBT-G as implemented at the Department of Personality Psychiatry has been very successful. In a recent study Kvarstein et al. (2014) compared data from the MBT programme, gathered since 2008 (n = 64 BPD patients), with the previous psychodynamic programme (n = 281 BPD patients). The MBT programme outperformed the psychodynamic programme on most outcome variables by effect sizes that were nearly twice as large (e.g., EZ 1.8 vs 0.9 for symptom distress). In the psychodynamic programme borderline patients had a very high dropout rate (42 %) during the first six months, and we were disturbed to find that they related this to their experiences with the group therapy (Hummelen et al., 2007). In the MBT programme these problems vanished, and the 6-month dropout rate was down to 5 %.

During recent years, courses in MBT-G have been arranged by the Norwegian Institute for Group Analysis (IGA) and the Norwegian Institute for Mentalization (IM). Training at the IGA used to consist of 10 days spread over two years, in concert with the block training courses in group analysis. Training at the IM consists of

8 days spread over one year, with no parallel self-experiential component. The candidates are supervised during training based upon video recordings of their ongoing groups. However, time does not allow for more than some short sequences of the respective groups. Consequently, there has been little knowledge about what might be the most important challenges when MBT-G was to be implemented in clinical practice at ordinary Mental Health Centers (MHC) in Norway. We thus were very curious when we succeeded to perform a video-based study of three consecutive sessions of a mentalization-based group at a MHC (Inderhaug & Karterud, 2015). Did the therapists succeed with their project and what were the main obstacles?

In the above mentioned study we found rather chaotic group processes, of a type which is well known from the literature (Pines, 1990; Marziali & Munroe-Blum, 1994; Hummelen, Wilberg & Karterud, 2007). The group was conducted by two therapists who had previous training in group analysis and MBT. We could observe that one of them (T1) consistently tried to apply MBT principles. However, the effect upon the group seemed minimal with respect to constructing scenarios that were useful for conjoint exploration and mentalizing. The therapists in the group we observed struggled to manage their authority in an efficient fashion, and also exhibited what we conceived as an exaggerated not-knowing attitude towards their therapeutic work. That is, the therapists were seen to adhere little to the item of managing authority, while the not-knowing stance was overplayed.

The therapists seemed to be trapped between two models. With one leg in each camp, they did not practice group analytic psychotherapy, nor did they practice MBT-G. Their dilemma possibly reflects the conceptual and therapeutic history of group analysis and MBT-G.

Concerning authority, Foulkes emphasised that the therapist(s) was not the leader of the group, but its conductor. He repeatedly argued against leadership in a traditional sense (Foulkes, 1964). The reasons were partly ideological, but mainly theoretical. We have to remember Foulkes' embeddedness in the antiauthoritarian Frankfurter School and the profound antiauthoritarian mentalities in Europe in the 1960s and 1970s. Perhaps more important was his theory of man: being profoundly social and "groupish" by nature, man would naturally strive for cooperation and group memberships. However, when hampered in his development, man would develop symptoms due to thwarted basic needs. In becoming member of a therapeutic group, the need for cooperation and group affiliation would be reactivated, accompanied with the individual's idiosyncratic ways of dealing with these needs. The symptoms would appear as group problems and the main task of the group analyst would be to assist the group in articulating these problems in the verbal discourse. Basically, these ideas are compatible with modern theories of the evolution of human thinking (Tomasello, 2014). Abstract and reflective social cognition are basically group phenomena which new members of the Homo sapiens group are predisposed to learn to become competent cooperative members of adult societies. Foulkes labelled the learning process "ego-training in action", while the corresponding MBT slogan is "the group as a training ground for mentalizing".

The overriding pragmatic question for both group analysis and MBT-G is now: What characterises a ground suited for proper training of the ego or mentalizing? Foulkes maintained that almost any kind of group (with respect to its members) conducted according to group analytic guidelines could become a proper training ground. I consider this view erroneous. To support this view, one should demonstrate empirically both high process qualities and favourable outcomes of groups composed of members who all share profound problems of social cognition/mentalizing, e.g., severe personality disorders. To my knowledge, there exists no report from group analytic practice which offers such support. Foulkes (and his generation of group analysts) seems to have underestimated the constituents of (successful) social cognition (Sharp et al., 2008). Successful social cognition (or good mentalizing abilities) is a late developmental achievement and dependent on the child being socialised by trustworthy adults and peers in safe situations. Furthermore, children seem to develop an "epistemic trust" when they encounter adults who perform a kind of "pedagogical stance", conveying basic properties and values of the social world (e.g., the inherent ethics of cooperative communication and concern for truth; Csibra & Gergely, 2009). Development of social cognition is thus dependent on a range of communicational qualities of the environment.

These prerequisites are likely to become violated when the communicational re-education take place in a group composed of personality disordered individuals who receive minimal instructions on how to proceed. Such experiments likely end up in disconnected speech and utterances, aborted stories conveying fragments of experience, emotional outbursts and activation of psychic equivalence, malign projective identifications, sequences of pseudomentalization, experiences of not being heard and respected, as well the hopelessness and disillusionment as demonstrated in several of the citations in the article of Inderhaug and Karterud (2015). Such situations call for therapists, not as conductors, but as competent leaders who model a kind of parental-like authority. This parental-like authority is less concerned with *what* is right or wrong, as *how* to reach truth about oneself and others. Philosophically, such an attitude is grounded in communicational ethics (e.g., Grice, 1991; Habermas, 1990) which concerns the implicit ethos of communication between humans, e.g., a wish for communication and conveying honest messages, a concern for truth, a respect for the dialog partner, active listening and an effort to understand the partner's mental state and point of view, etc. This kind of communication does not come by nature. It is hard won achievements of cultural (group) evolution. The concept of mentalizing stance belongs to this tradition of ideas.

Although communicational ethics is a cultural (group) product, being legitimised and sanctioned by cultural codes and practices, the pragmatics of communication is most often discussed with references to a two-person kind of dialogue ("I – Thou"). When it comes to group situations things get complicated, and culture has invented a series of procedures for securing rational reasoning. There is an implicit and explicit cultural knowledge ("common ground") that group situations easily activate mental phenomena that run counter to rationality. The pioneering work of Bion

(1961) conceptualised these difficulties in the basic assumption theory, contending that rationality was a property of the "work group", while pre-mentalistic cognition flourished in the "basic assumption group". The position of group analysis has been to abolish ordinary procedures for group cooperation, e.g., by encouraging free group associations. This would ultimately liberate the group from harsh superego control and rigid cultural artefacts.. MBT-G, on the other hand, maintains that, depending on the group member's level of personality functioning, a certain communicational structure is necessary for reason to survive and thrive. This requires leadership. The therapists must uphold a communicational ideal, to model it, strive for it, defend it, explicate its *raison d'etre*, and try to recruit other group members so that the group self becomes embodied not merely by the therapists, but by other group members as well (Karterud, 1998). There is a lot of "knowing" embedded in this undertaking with respect to communicational processes and how to intervene, e.g., how to identify poor versus good mentalizing and their effects on the group process. It is easy to lose this knowledge when being bombarded by projective identifications. It is all the more important therefore, that the therapist pair is firmly grounded in the ethos of their therapeutic project.

According to this logic, the not-knowing stance comes second to communicational structuring. In order to train in mentalizing, in a more limited sense, one need scenes (either in the group, or in the narrative) with protagonists in time-sequential events. Through such scenes group members can imaginatively explore mental states, their intersubjective connectedness, contextual dependency and implications for the subject(s) who "own" the scenes. There is in such scenes that the therapists have to refrain from the temptation to "know" the "hidden" motives behind the transactions, and to facilitate the group member's open-minded exploration of minds.

Basically, the idea is that by the individual group members striving to become a member of the mentalizing group self, i.e. the work group aspect of the group, one has to develop one's social cognition (Karterud & Stone, 2003). Or phrased in another way: the development of social cognition (narration, attention, focusing, inhibitory control, affect consciousness, metacognition, mentalizing, integration, etc.) is likely to be a result of one's efforts to become a member of the group self. This logic is supported by modern theories of evolution of thinking, self-consciousness and culture (Bogdan, 2010; Tomasello, 2014).

The findings of our companion study (Inderhaug & Karterud, 2015) illustrate some difficulties therapists encounter when trying to establish themselves as leaders for a certain communicational structure when the group members easily resort to primitive modes of mentalizing. The therapists in this study were overheard, not paid attention to, interrupted, and at times ridiculed. As explained in previous paragraphs, no development of social cognition can take place in such a discourse. The therapists were vaguely aware of the discrepancies between their therapeutic ideals and the chaotic group discourse. However, they feared aggressive outbursts in the group, felt helpless when they experienced the absence of therapeutic alliance, and lost confidence in MBT-G principles. Nevertheless, they tried to practice a kind of not-knowing stance. However, these attempts failed since the structure could not capture and contain adequate scenes long enough for joint exploration to take place. The result was pseudomentalization. Phrased in an object-relational language, many of the therapist's difficulties can be conceived as countertransference strategies for coping with severe "attacks on linking" (Bion, 1970). Bion coined this term as a slogan for destructive mental processes of non-integration and resistance towards construction of meaning. Such attacks are as expected in groups with borderline patients. In order to deal with attacks of this magnitude (augmented by group processes), there is an obvious need for professional support and supervisory assistance. The lack of such support may be one explanation why MBT-G which has proved very efficient in an academic/university setting with a high professional standard (Kvarstein et al., 2014), failed to do so in an ordinary MHC. Supervisory services thus have to be strengthened for MBT-G. There already exist in Norway a MBT quality assurance laboratory who performs such services for individual MBT. This year we hope to extend those services to include also MBT-G. There is also an obvious need to publish qualitative studies on successful MBT-G. By comparing successful and failed attempts at practicing MBT-G we might obtain more knowledge about the pragmatics of communication within this particular type of group discourse. Such studies are under way.

References

Bales, D., van Beek, N., Smits, M., Willemsen, S., Bussbach, J. J. V., Verheul, R. & Andrea, H. (2012). Treatment outcome of 18-month, day hospital mentalization-based treatment (MBT) in patients with severe borderline personality disorder in the Netherlands. *Journal of Personality Disorders*, 26(4): 568–582.

Bateman, A. & Fonagy, P. (2001). Treatment of borderline personality disorder with psychoanalytically oriented partial hospitalization: An 18-month follow-up. *American Journal of Psychiatry*, 158: 36–42.

Bateman, A. & Fonagy, P. (2009). Randomized controlled trial of outpatient mentalization-based treatment versus structured clinical management for borderline personality disorder. *American Journal of Psychiatry*, 166: 1355–1364.

Bateman, A. W. & Fonagy, P. (2004). *Psychotherapy for Borderline Personality Disorder. Mentalization-based Treatment*. Oxford: Oxford University Press.

Bateman, A. W. & Fonagy, P. (2006a). *Mentalization Based Treatment for Borderline Personality Disorder: A Practical Guide*. Oxford: Oxford University Press.

Bateman, A. W. & Fonagy, P. (2006b). Mentalizing and borderline personality disorder. In J. G. Allen & P. Fonagy (Eds.), *Handbook of Mentalization-based Treatment*. West Sussex: Wiley.

Bion, W. R. (1961). *Experiences in Groups*. London: Tavistock Publications.

Bion, W. R. (1970). *Attention and Interpretation*. London: Tavistock Publications.

Bogdan, R. J. (2010). *Our Own Minds. Sociocultural Grounds for Self-consciousness*. London: The MIT Press.

Cibra, G. & Gergely, G. (2009). Natural pedagogy. *Trends in Cognitive Science,* 13(4): 148–153.

Farrell, J. M. & Shaw, I. A. (2012). *Group Schema Therapy for Borderline Personality Disorder.* West Sussex: Wiley-Blackwell.

Fonagy, P., Bateman, A. & Bateman, A. (2011). The widening scope of mentalizing: A discussion. *Psychology and Psychotherapy: Theory, Research and Practice,* 84: 98–110.

Foulkes, S. H. (1964). *Therapeutic Group-analysis.* London: G. Allen and Unwin Ltd.

Grice, P. (1991). *Studies in the Way of Words.* London: Harvard University Press.

Habermas, J. (1990). *Moral Consciousness and Communicative Action.* Cambridge: Polity Press.

Hummelen, B., Wilberg, T. & Karterud, S. (2007). Interviews of female patients with borderline personality disorder who dropped out of group psychotherapy. *International Journal of Group Psychotherapy,* 57(1): 67–91.

Inderhaug, T. S. & Karterud, S. (2015). A qualitative study of a mentalization-based group for borderline patients. *Group Analysis*, 48(2): 341–349.

Karterud, S. (1998). The group self, empathy, intersubjectivity and hermeneutics. A group analytic perspective. In I. Harwood & M. Pines (Eds.), *Self Experiences in Group. Intersubjective and Self Psychological Pathways to Human Understanding.* London: Jessica Kingsley Publishers.

Karterud, S. (2011). Constructing and mentalizing the matrix. *Group Analysis,* 44(4): 1–17.

Karterud, S. (2012). *Manual for mentaliseringbasert gruppeterapi (MBT-G).* Oslo: Gyldendal Akademisk.

Karterud, S. & Stone, W. N. (2003). The group self: A neglected aspect of group psychotherapy. *Group Analysis,* 36(1): 7–22.

Karterud, S. & Wilberg, T. (2007). From general day hospital treatment to specialized treatment programs. *International Review of Psychiatry,* 19(1): 39–49.

Karterud, S. & Bateman, A. (2010). *Manual for mentaliseringbasert terapi (MBT) og MBT vurderingsskala. Versjon individualterapi.* Oslo: Gyldendal Akademisk.

Karterud, S. & Bateman, A. (2011). Group therapy techniques. In P. Fonagy & A. Bateman (Eds.), *Mentalizing in Mental Health Practice.* Washington: American Psychiatric Press.

Karterud, S., Pedersen, G., Johansen, M. S., Johansen, P., Schlüter, C., Engen, M., Wilberg, T., Urnes, Ø. & Bateman, A. (2013). The mentalization-based treatment adherence and competence scale (MBT-ACS): Development, structure and reliability. *Psychotherapy Research,* 23(6): 674–698.

Kvarstein, E., Pedersen, G., Urnes, Ø., Hummelen, B., Wilberg, T. & Karterud, S. (2014). Changing from a traditional psychodynamic treatment program to mentalization-based treatment for patients with borderline personality disorder. Does it make a difference? *Psychology and Psychotherapy: Theory, Research and Practice.* DOI: 10.1111/papr.12036

Linehan, M. M. (1993). *Skills Training Manual for Treating Borderline Personality Disorder.* New York: The Guilford Press.

Luborsky, L. & Barber, J. P. (1993). Benefits of adherence to psychotherapy manuals, and where to get them. In N. E. Miller, L. E. Luborsky, J. P. Barber, & J. P. Docherty (Eds.), *Psychodynamic Treatment Research: A Handbook for Clinical Practice* (pp. 211–226). New York: Basic Books.

Marsiali, E. & Munroe-Blum, H. (1994). *Interpersonal Group Psychotherapy for Borderline Personality Disorder.* New York: Basic Books.

Pines, M. (1990). Group analytic psychotherapy and the borderline patient. In B. E. Roth, W. N. Stone, & H. D. (Eds.), *The Difficult Patient in Group*. Madison: International Universities Press.

Rossouw, T. & Fonagy, P. (2012). Mentalization-based treatment for self-harm in adolescents: A randomized controlled trial. , 51(12): 1304–1313.

Roth, B. E., Stone, W. N. & Kibel, H. D. (Eds.) (1990). *The Difficult Patient in Group*. Madison: International Universities Press.

Rutan, S. C., Stone, W. N. & Shay, J. J. (2007). *Psychodynamic Group Psychotherapy*. New York: The Guilford Press.

Sharp, C., Fonagy, P. & Goodyer, I (Eds.) (2008). *Social Cognition and Developmental Psychopathology*. Oxford: Oxford University Press.

Tomasello, M. (2014). *A Natural History of Human Thinking*. London: Harvard University Press.

Yalom, I. D. & Leszcz, M. (2005). *The Theory and Practice of Group Psychotherapy*. New York: Basic Books.

Chapter 7

A comparative study of mentalization-based versus psychodynamic group therapy

Jens Kalleklev and Sigmund Karterud

Abstract

Aims: The purpose of this study was to investigate how mentalization-based group therapy (MBT-G) for patients with borderline personality disorder is both different and similar to a more traditional psychodynamic group psychotherapy approach.

Material and methods: The study is a comparative case-study examining a representative clinical example of MBT-G and a supposedly representative clinical example of a psychodynamic group (PDG). Both groups were composed mainly of patients with borderline personality disorder. The study used a mixed methodological approach with quantitative research methods, including MBT-G Adherence and Quality Scale and Reflective Functioning Scale (RF-scale), and qualitative content analysis.

Results: 1) MBT-G therapists had a consistently higher focus on mental states. This was reflected both in the significantly higher intervention frequency (294 in the MBT group vs. 130 in the PDG), and in the higher proportion of theoretically assumed mentalizing-promoting interventions (228 vs. 16 interventions adhering to MBT-G-ASQ). 2) Therapists from both groups actively structured the sessions, but the MBT group more explicitly discussed whether a topic should or should not be put on the agenda. 3) RF increased more pronounced during the sequences in the MBT group than in the PDG. 4) Interventions with "demand" characteristics played an important role in the development of the mentalizing group discourse.

Conclusion: Despite superficial similarities between the approaches, differences in choice of therapeutic focus and consistency suggest that the two methods engage patients in different therapy processes. Due to the study's limited population, the generalizability of the results is uncertain.

DOI: 10.4324/9781003625810-7

Introduction

Mentalization-based treatment (MBT) belongs to the psychodynamic tradition. The first trial (Bateman & Fonagy, 1999) even used the phrase "psychoanalytic day hospital". The main target for MBT, borderline personality disorder, is conceptualised as an attachment-, relational- and self-disorder with affect regulation and mentalizing deficits (Bateman & Fonagy, 2006). MBT is a conjoint kind of treatment, composed of individual and group therapies. The dynamic group component developed from a British group analytic/psychodynamic group therapy matrix. How far is modern mentalization-based group therapy (MBT-G) from its siblings?

The topic has been discussed in previous issues of *Group Analysis* (Potthoff & Moini-Afchari 2014). Pothoff and Moini-Afchari (2014) writes that, on the one hand it has been maintained that MBT-G represents a paradigm shift in the way of conducting group therapy and that MBT-G could replace traditional group analysis (Schultz-Venrath, 2010). Others have been more sceptical and doubted that MBT-G offers anything new (Rudolf, 2006), and argued that MBT and psychoanalytic-interactional approaches are very similar and pointed out that the traditional repertoire has always included interventions that intend to foster mentalizing. These are clarification (Glover, 1955), mirroring (Kohut, 1983; Winnicott, 1971) and detailed inquiry (Sullivan, 1954) to name a few.

Already in the early development of group analysis, Foulkes (1964) emphasised the unique potential groups had to mirror self-states, object relations, and emotions, which he gives priority in his communication theory (Potthoff & Moini-Afchari 2014). Also, others have pointed to the dangers of malicious, false mirroring ("malignant mirroring"), e.g., when a group member feels consistently misunderstood or overlooked (Zinkin, 1992). These and other challenges with borderline patients in psychodynamic group therapy has long been known, e.g., through descriptions of how projective identification can dominate in groups of this population (Zender, 1991). As a leader in such groups, one is therefore constantly confronted with complications that quickly need to be cleared up and resolved. One has, therefore, realised that it would be counter-productive to keep an attitude of evenly suspended attention in such situations, which is generally recommended in conventional group analytical techniques (Foulkes, 1964; Potthoff & Moini-Afchari 2014). One finds, therefore, that within recent group analytical thinking, it is expected that the BDP-patients' typical structural weakness sometimes will require more intensive work individually, which in periods might affect the free flow of group processes (Berghaus & Potthoff, 2009).

The above-mentioned considerations are mainly based upon clinical reports and risk being speculative. We lack empirical studies, which can enlighten the topic. In this article, we present a relevant clinical study. We have compared, head on, a MBT group session (from 2014) with a psychodynamic group session (from

2006). Both groups were conducted at the same clinical department, with the same type of clientele, but at different periods of time, which hosted different treatment regimes. In what respects are these groups similar or different? Answers to these questions may be helpful in explicating the nature of these groups, and what kind of processes they elicit in their members. Thus, answers may be useful for a more enlightened discussion of how groups should be designed for different purposes. E.g., should group analysis adopt elements from MBT-G when the patient population is predominantly personality disorders? And what elements should those be?

Material and methods

The material for this study was two group therapy sessions conducted at the Department of Personality Psychiatry, Oslo University Hospital. The first group session, recorded on 13 August 2006, was from an outpatient group, which served as continuation treatment after an initial short-term day hospital phase. The treatment ideology was psychodynamic, integrating object-relations theory and self-psychology, and treatment technique was leaning on (modified) group analytic psychotherapy. We label this group the "psychodynamic group" (PDG). The two therapists were both qualified group analysts, a psychiatrist and a clinical social worker. All patients had a PD diagnosis, most often of cluster B (borderline) type. The patients ought to be considerably affected (symptomatically and functionally) in order to receive this treatment. The group was video recorded as part of the Ullevål Personality Project (UPP). The results of this treatment were moderately good, as reported in several follow up studies (Gullestad, Wilberg, Klungsøyr, Urnes, & Karterud, 2012; Antonsen et al., 2014).

This way of organizing and doing treatment for patients with PD´s was terminated in 2008 when the whole department underwent a radical reorientation and adopted MBT as its principal approach. The second group was recorded on 21 January 2014 and was part of this new MBT intensive outpatient program. One of the two therapists was a qualified group analyst and trained in MBT. The other therapist was a psychiatric resident with no formal group or MBT training. The patients were similar to those in 2006, possibly with some more borderline features. The results of this treatment have been reported by Kvarstein et al. (2014) and were found to be very good, with effect sizes that were nearly twice as high as the psychodynamic program.

Patients in both groups gave their written informed consent which was approved by the regional ethics committee and the patient ombudsman at Oslo University Hospital (OUS).

The methods for the study were both quantitative and qualitative. Both groups were carefully transcribed by the first author and both groups were rated according to the MBT-G Adherence and Quality Scale (MBT-G-AQS) by the Norwegian MBT laboratory (www.youtube.com/watch?v=hddIUpUOZdw) (Karterud, 2015). In brief, the scale consists of nine group-specific items of MBT-G and ten general items for MBT (which are similar to items in the MBT individual therapy scale). All therapist interventions are rated according to the MBT-G-AQS, for adherence/frequency as well as quality. Interventions that do not comply with any of the items do not receive any rating. There is also given an overall rating for the session as a whole. It was obvious from the outset that the MBT group would receive a higher adherence score than the PDG. However, it was expected that also the PDG would contain interventions that promoted mentalization, e.g., by focus on affects and reflections on affects.

Complementing the analysis of mentalizing content in the groups, all patient statement were rated according to the Reflective Function Scale (RF-scale) (Fonagy, Target, Steele, & Steele, 1998). The RF-scores represent the extent to which the interviewee in an Adult Attachment Interview (AAI) address and elaborate on mental states in their responses (Hesse, 2008). Reflection on higher mentalizing levels involves adopting a tentative approach that seeks to understand own and others' feelings, thoughts and behaviour from different perspectives. The opposite is not to relate events and behavioural expressions to internal mental states. Responses are graded on a Likert-scale where scores from -1 to 3 is interpreted as negative to limited RF, and scores of 5 to 9 as moderate to high RF. The mean response for a normal population to AAI has been shown to be around 5 (Fonagy et al., 1996; Pedersen, Lunn, Katznelson, & Poulsen, 2012). Recent research has shown that MBT adherence and competence predicts higher session RF among patients, even when controlling for pre-treatment RF (Møller et al., 2016).

In AAI, only the patients' responses to challenging questions (demand questions) are rated by the RF scale. Demand questions address the patients directly about what they feel and think about themselves and their attachment figures. As opposed to permit questions, which are more open and less activating, demand questions often challenge the mentalizing ability by arousing more affect, due to an activated attachment system (Fonagy et al., 1998; Hesse, 2008). Examples of questions from AAI may be "why do you think your parents did this?" or "do you think they realized you felt rejected?". A characteristic of such "demand questions" is that they require a mentalizing response, while "permit questions" do not. Recent research has showed that interventions directed toward exploring mental states predicts higher RF of subsequent patient responses (Møller et al., 2016). In our study, such interventions were coded as demand interventions. Questions that did not involve intentional/motivational mental states were coded as permit interventions. The RF ratings in this study were done by the first author, consulting with the second author.

When it comes to processing the RF scores, we looked at the RF ratings chronologically and patient wise. Our intention was to track variations in RF level as the therapeutic dialogue unfolded over time, and possibly noting important points of significant change. A point of interest, was to identify if certain therapist interventions (e.g. demand or permit) played a role in facilitating RF change more than others.

Our analysis was also completed with an extended qualitative approach, where we aimed at developing a descriptive account of the content unfolding in the groups (Merriam, 1988). This phase endeavoured to be both exploratory and theory-driven, where MBT theory and other group therapy theory served as an organizing principle (Lincoln & Guba, 1985).

Results

Therapist interventions

A simple counting of therapist interventions clearly differentiated the groups. In the MBT group, there were 294 therapist interventions versus 130 interventions in the PDG. It is not surprising that MBT therapist are more active than the PDG therapists. However, Table 7.1 reveals differences which are larger than we expected. Only 16 of the 130 interventions in the PDG complied with the MBT items, compared to 228 of 294 interventions in the MBT group. *This indicates that these therapists actually did quite different things.* We had expected that also therapists

Table 7.1 Frequency of therapist's interventions in psychodynamic versus mentalization-based group therapy

MBT-G-ACS items	*Frequency in PDF*	*Frequency MBT-G*
1. Handling of group boundaries	2	5
2. Regulating group phases	1	15
3. Initiative and implementation of turn-taking	0	12
4. Engagement of group members in mentalizing external events	0	13
5. Identification and mentalizing events in the group	0	35
6. Caring for the group and each member. (only scored for quality)	-	-
7. Displaying authority. (only scored for quality)	-	-
8. Encouraging relevant group as whole discussions	0	5
9. Cooperation with co-therapist	1	1
10. Engagement, interest and warm (only scored for quality)	-	-
11. Exploration, curiosity and not-knowing stance	6	25
12. Challenging unwarranted beliefs	0	16
13. Regulation of arousal	1	9
14. Rewarding good mentalizing	0	4
15. Handling pretend mode	1	11
16. Handling psychic equivalence	0	0
17. Focus on affects	3	43
18. Use of stop and rewind	0	0
19. Focus on the relationship between therapists and patients	1	34

in the PDG would to a larger extent focus on affects, explore with a not-knowing stance and engage patients in mentalizing external and internal group events. They did not. They did different things.

MBT-G adherence and quality rating scale

The overall rating of the MBT group was 7 on adherence and 6 on quality. In other words, the MBT- group was conducted in a high degree of accordance with the manual. The PDG was given an overall score of 1 for adherence and 2 for quality. These overall ratings indicate large differences between the groups.

Description of the sequences

Our analysis revealed that the breakup of the group sessions in sequences made them especially suitable for comparison. The sequences were characterised by a continuous focus on a theme or a person. Both groups consisted of a total of five sequences. In the MBT-G group, this included an opening agenda setting, and a closing sequence. The PDG had only therapeutic sequences, i.e. there were no discussions whether a topic should or should not be put on the agenda. Instead, the participants themselves often spontaneously initiated sequences, or were invited in by the therapists along the way. In contrast, the structuring in the MBT group were often explicitly discussed. Curiously, some of the MBT patients demonstrated limited motivation about addressing the topics that were put on the agenda. However, their interest seemed to grow in the course of the sessions. Both groups also contained several smaller in-between exchanges with other patients touching on the same or related themes. These additions were in varying degree either contributing to or derailing from the perceived therapeutic focus. It was distinctive for the MBT group that these events were a subject for group discussions. A short summary of each sequence is provided below.

Sequences from the MBT-group

Opening sequence (duration 5 minutes). A short recap on events and themes touched upon in the last meeting were discussed, as well as inviting each patient to share their thoughts for new topics on today's agenda. A total of four themes were agreed on (but only three were addressed).

Clinical sequence 1 (duration 35 minutes). This is the main sequence in the group, and the person in centre is patient L, a woman in her 30s. She started out in a nonmentalizing manner and described herself as empty, having nothing to talk about. This sequence has been described in detail (verbatim) in a companion article (Karterud, 2018), and demonstrates how she, through a series of challenging interventions from the therapists, gradually recovers her mentalizing abilities and gets involved in a complex and highly meaningful interaction with her fellow group mates around important borderline dynamics.

Clinical sequence 2 (duration 20 minutes). Here, patient A, also a woman in her thirties, requested a discussion of her therapy termination. She argued that she felt "completely mentalized" and referred to other people's opinions that she is ready to move on. This suggests a pseudomentalizing level of functioning (RF=1–3). In the first half of the sequence, she remains stagnant in terms of RF, and the rest of the group seems quite aloof (some even fronting scepticism) about having an opinion about the subject. However, after having negotiated an agreement, patient A expresses relief and shares details about how she succeeded in her therapy process, exemplified through accounts of how her perspective has changed. She now experience having a choice in situations, where she before felt trapped. Seeing more clearly the destructiveness of her previous escapism, has made it a non-applicable option. Also, admitting the inevitability of sporadically rebounds of intense feelings of jealousy, she demonstrated acceptance and coping strategies, which made her come across as convincingly matured. In this second half of the sequence, her RF rose to about 5, and the group climate transformed from scepticism and non-involvement to highly engaged with questions and comments. This transformation demonstrates a classic example of installation of hope (Yalom & Lesczc, 2005).

Clinical sequence 3 (duration 25 minutes). The last therapy sequence concerned patient S' (a woman in her 20s) repeated trouble with remembering what transpired in previous sessions. The subject was suggested by the therapists, and despite her initial agreement to look at it, patient S appeared defensive and non-involved. Her dismissive stance "what do you want me to say about that?!", implies a non-mentalizing level (RF=0). This created immediately a deadlock, but the therapists successfully opened space for other group members to reflect and explore the phenomenon. S, however, demonstrated no reflection involving mental states. The group effort also included a fruitful mentalizing discussion about derailing from the agreed upon focus. Ironically, however, the therapist's efforts to engage S with challenging (demand) interventions, e.g., commenting on her conspicuous non-involvement in the subject, failed to extract a response, as other group members derailed by offering advice or throwing humorous remarks.

Closing sequence. The remaining few minutes of the session were devoted to an evaluation of the meeting and mapped out topics needed to be addressed in a subsequent session.

Sequences from the PDG

Clinical sequence 1 (duration 15 minutes). Patient C, a woman in her 30s, started out spontaneously, expressing that she suddenly had become "superdepressed and pissed" lately. Queried about the nature of the depression, C just denoted it as "ordinary", suggesting a low level of mentalization (RF=1-3). When mirrored in her quick answers, she assured her truthfulness. The following exploration of events that may have triggered the depression, eventually revealed that she also had become shier lately, which caused her irritation (slightly rise of RF). She later linked her shyness to a lack of energy to celebrate her birthday the way she normally would. The group's exploration touched upon mental states, but the mentalizing focus was quickly redirected to supportive statements or clarification of events, leading her to link the lack of energy to her work disability. C's quick answers were also mirrored a second time and led to C explaining that she practiced being honest and direct, a trait her boyfriend had encouraged. She admitted also that this probably made her depleted of energy, but there was no reference to mental states in explaining her behaviour. In summary, the pseudomentalizing, which dominated the sequence, was not resolved, and even possibly strengthened by surprisingly supportive interventions like "I believe you will find the answers in yourself", etc.

Clinical sequence 2 (duration 5 minutes). This sequence contained for the most part a news report from patient E, a woman in her 20s, who had finally graduated as a nurse, and had got a half time job in a hospital. The group expressed happiness on her behalf and were curious to hear details about the situation. About the prospects of managing the new employment, she revealed that she had been open about her mental problems to her boss, who responded understandingly. Her therapy termination was also discussed. This sequence operated at a fairly low mentalizing level (RF=1-3), and the therapist interventions and other patient comments were primarily supportive and/or clarifying in nature, with examples like "Wow, you got the job even before you received the results from the exam!" or "So your economic situation will be better now?".

Clinical sequence 3 (duration 25 minutes). This sequence started by one of the therapists noticing on the shopping bags patient F, a woman in her late 20s, brought into the session, and wondering about the underlying motive (demand question). In response, F explained how she grabbed a rare opportunity to treat herself with something extra, as she had inherited some money. However, spending money triggers a continuous conflict concerning economical dependency to her parents. The group then engaged in exploring and clarifying her economic problems. At one point, patient C gives F a compliment on her new dress and haircut. Sometime later, C confronted F and asked if she reacted fearfully to her compliment. F denied it, declaring that she thought she had mastered how to say thank you. C tentatively links the reaction to F's body image, but the beginning mentalizing focus disappeared quickly in favour of returning to the former focus on how to manage her economy. The root of the problem crystallized as a distrust of her abilities to care for herself. Summarized, again the dominating pseudomentalizing mode was not adequately challenged, and again seemed reinforced by the supportive interventional style of both the therapists and the group.

Clinical *sequence 4 (duration 40 minutes).* Here, patient A, a woman in her early 20s, started out exclaiming that "everything is shit". Invited to explore the problem, she rejected, claiming she didn't want to cry. Shifting the focus on to her background, she soon got overwhelmed again and started to denigrate herself as hopeless in handling irritating schoolmates and invading neighbours. She also described how she acts out in self-destructive ways by, i.e. eating junk food (she is a vegetarian). Her mentalizing mode is psychic equivalence (RF=1). Then, patient F entered and empathically shared her experience of recognizing A's situation, as she herself have had similar experiences. This initiated a group process of receiving and processing the emotional communication from A without being overwhelmed by it, and then processing it and communicating back an understanding and recognition without necessarily suggesting any action. This sequence might be labelled a classic example of "containing" (Bion, 1970). A bit later, A, seemed somewhat more able to share stressful life experiences with drug abuse, and losing her boyfriend, her job and her social network. Later, one of the therapists mirrored A's wish to maintain boundaries towards others (neighbours etc.), but this caused A to regress and feel like a loser. Again, patient F, returned to contain her sense of hopelessness and frustration. Despite the prevalence of psychic equivalence (RF= 1-3), the containing part seemed to have some impact on A's ability to process emotions and thoughts concerning her situation.

Clinical sequence 5 (duration 3 minutes). The session concludes with a supportive «check-out» on patient B, a man about 30 years. The focus was on how he was doing after the session last week, and how he will manage this time.

Further observations from the sessions

Across both groups, the mentalizing level in the dialogues were generally very low at the beginning of the sequences (RF =1-3). In general, patients described situations and events, rather than feelings and mental states. However, the range of RF in the MBT group span from 1 to 7, while the PDG ranged between 1 to 5. Two of the sequences (sequence 1 and 2) in the MBT group showed a clear, gradual increase in RF. In the remaining sequences (both the MBT-group and the PDG), the pattern was less systematic and could vary slightly up and down without any clear direction, sometimes at a fairly constant level, with occasional highs or lows.

More specifically, the RF boost witnessed in the mentioned MBT-G sequences, fell in a context of a series of challenging therapist interventions (demand questions), which represented a stabilization of the therapeutic focus and its mentalizing quality over a considerable timespan. The sequence of patient L in the MBT group (presented in the companion article), illustrates this phenomenon. Being unable to respond satisfactory to the initial demand intervention, L gradually turned her attention inward, in line with the demands of the intervention – demands that were not abandoned but rather reformulated again and again, until a more satisfactory answer was produced. However, the process was not a smooth road and included periods where the dialogue came to a standstill or was going in circles, at times when the specifics of the demand questions were not yet answered satisfactorily. In this void, both therapists and participants became engaged in helping to fill in the "missing pieces" and often arrived at a more elaborated mentalizing account of the problem. Gradually, this seemed to help break the entrenched pre-mentalizing habitual thinking (pseudomentalizing) of the patient in focus.

In contrast, the PDG group did not demonstrate such patterns with a therapeutic focus on demand questions. If posed, the demand questions (or other interventions that were identified through the MBT-G-ASQ), were not followed up by therapists or were somehow diverted by fellow group members imposing an alternative route of exploration. Clearly, this particular mentalizing-promoting approach was not a part of the PDG strategy. Rather, as seen in patient F's sequence, the sporadic mentalizing therapeutic foci were quickly abandoned for the benefit of other foci. Instead of exploring the underlying mental states leading to her reaction, the dialogue was transformed into a more general exploration of how to accept compliments. Overall, the intervention strategy in the PDG was predominantly more supportively oriented than challenging.

Discussion

The main findings from the study were that:

1) MBT-G therapists had a consistently higher focus on mental states and emotions. This was reflected both in the significantly higher intervention frequency (294 in the MBT group vs. 130 in the PDG), and in the higher proportion of theoretically assumed mentalizing-promoting interventions (228 vs. 16 MBT-G-ASQ rated interventions).
2) Therapists from both groups actively structured the sessions, but the MBT group more explicitly discussed whether a topic should or should not be put on the agenda.
3) RF increased more pronounced during the sequences in the MBT group than in the PDG.
4) Interventions with "demand" characteristics played an important role in the development of the mentalizing group discourse.

In the following, we will discuss these results in more detail.

1. Focus on mental states

The consistent focus on mental states and emotions (228 of 294 interventions), which we found in the MBT-G, but not in the PDG group, suggests that the MBT-G therapists and the PDG therapists did different things. A high frequency of mentalizing interventions is to be expected in MBT-G, but we had also expected a larger proportion of mentalizing interventions in the PDG. In fact, according to the MBT-G-ASQ, the mentalizing focus in the PDG was almost absent (only in 16 of 130 interventions).

However, this dramatic difference should be somewhat moderated, as a high proportion of the PDG interventions were clarifying in nature. According to Kernberg (1984), clarifying the course of events, makes it possible to reconsider the "true" nature of events, which may foster the patient's ability to perceive, interpret, remember, think, consider, decide and then act appropriately in the face of a real-life problem. Thus, clarification implies mentalizing promoting processes, although the exact relationship to MBT interventions is somewhat complex. We find remnants of clarification in item 11 (exploration, curiosity and not-knowing stance) of the MBT-G-ASQ (Karterud, 2015) and item 16 (therapists checking out their understanding with the patients) of the MBT-I-ASQ (Karterud & Bateman, 2011), but these interventions are still more specifically directed at mental states, rather than aiming for clarity on a more general level. Another common denominator with MBT interventions is relying on asking questions, as opposed to presenting interpretations. This way, therapists avoid adopting an expert role and may point to contradictions or ambiguities in the patient's narrative in a more tentative way. Moreover, rather than giving the missing pieces, the therapist lets the patient himself make the effort to put the pieces together. In both MBT-G and supportive variants of psychodynamic therapy, this is considered useful, as it helps build ego-strength or mentalizing ability in the patient herself respectively (as opposed to becoming dependent on the therapist's "expert knowledge") (Karterud, 1999; Lorentzen, 2014).

There were also other events in the PDG group stemming from patient activity, which may have contributed to mentalization-relevant group processes. An example is the containment episode, which potentially helped restore the capacity to think under activation of strong negative emotions (Bion, 1970).

Summarized, it seems an important difference between the methods concerning what content the therapists are actively addressing. On a superficial level, these differences may be overlooked, conveying the impression of similarity between these different group modes. Both groups contained 6-7 similar patients sitting in a circle with two therapists who tried to stimulate collective reflections on their life experiences. However, the lack of a consistent focus on mental states in the PDG suggests that we are talking about different therapeutic purposes and different therapeutic processes.

2. Structuring of the group

Compared to the MBT group, the relatively low intervention frequency, and the lack of an opening agenda setting, might facilitate the PDG group process towards letting it express itself spontaneously. This is thought to help unconscious interactional patterns emerge, which thereby becomes available for clarification and interpretation (Karterud, 1999; Lorentzen, 2014). This is basically seen as a healthy part of the group process signalling growing patient autonomy (Lorentzen, 2014). According to psychodynamic group therapy theory, the high therapist activity we saw in the MBT-group could possibly be seen as disturbance of an "open-ended" process, which is preferably to be expressed without too much intervention or predefined goals (Foulkes, 1964). Also traditionally, setting an agenda at the start of the meeting is not recommended, as it is thought to encourage intellectualization rather than free floating association and interaction (Karterud, 1999).

However, compared to traditional group analytic therapy, the PDG demonstrated more structuring of the therapy process than we had expected. This coincide with more supportive-oriented approaches, where therapists are taking greater responsibility to include participants, who for various reasons remain passive (Lorentzen, 2014). With borderline patients, this strategy may help avoiding group members feel misunderstood or overlooked (Zinkin, 1992). In this way, the PDG contained a mixture of patients spontaneously putting themselves on the agenda (free associating), and therapists structuring through addressing patients directly with questions about specific topics. As a result, this created a structure where "everybody" got their turn, rather similar to the pattern of sequences we found in the MBT-group. However, in the PDG there was no explicit discussion about what should be put on the agenda or not. *Therefore, the difference between the groups was not so much about having a turn-taking structure or not, but rather about the degree of explicitness in discussing whom and what these turns should be about.*

3. RF change

The greater increase in RF scores in the MBT-G group may not be surprising, since stimulating mentalization is the primary goal of MBT. Nevertheless, to our knowledge there exist no previous studies that have explored this particular topic in group therapy. Therefore, the finding is not trivial, as it supports basic assumptions about the causal mechanisms of MBT-G. Speaking conversely, an absence of such a correlation between mentalizing intervention and RF in patient responses could have raised doubts about the MBT-G's suitability to build mentalization ability. However, this finding is not very robust. There was no reliability check on the ratings of patients' RF scores. The similar findings from individual MBT are more substantial (Möller et al., 2016). Interestingly, the low RF levels at the start of each sequence indicate that there is no automaticity in establishing a mentalizing discourse. Taking into account that the members of the MBT group also had completed a psychoeducational MBT group, received parallel individual MBT sessions, and had frequently been exposed to a mentalizing group discourse, suggest that a mentalizing group dialogue is quite counterintuitive and requires great effort to achieve for this group of patients (patients with BPD), which is especially prone to habitual prementalistic modes of thinking and relating (Bateman & Fonagy, 2004). To counteract this tendency, reminding the patients of the purpose of (MBT) group psychotherapy, should possibly be a routine requirement.

4. Role of demand interventions in group psychotherapy

Identifying interventions and strategies for maximizing mentalizing in groups are important topics for further developments in group psychotherapy. In this study, demand interventions emerged as a candidate factor in facilitating mentalizing. Possibly, it may be that the mentalizing clarity of demand interventions more effectively guides patients into a mentalizing mindset. The specificity of these questions, also make it more conspicuously if patients fail to respond to them. In response to permit interventions, which involves querying in a more open manner, patients may more easily respond in avoiding or habitual ways, without involving mental states, and without it being regarded defensive by the rest of the group. As we saw from the sequence of patient L in the MBT group (described in the companion article), the demand questions were already touched upon in the opening sequence and were kept in focus with some variation throughout the whole sequence. This seemed to trigger the patient, either due to perceived external pressure from the group or from internal dissonance, to fill the gap between her habitual answers and the potential implicit in the questions. In other words, demand interventions may activate a motive to find the "missing pieces", thereby initiating increased mentalizing effort. *A key point of understanding, we believe, is that the possible transformative power of these interventions not only lies in the demand characteristics, but also in the painstaking efforts to keep them in focus over a time span.* Possibly, this combination pays off and evolves the discourse further, and may even help dissolve standstills or deadlocking, due to a growing discontent with the limitations of quick, habitual, pseudomentalizing answers. In this way, the above-mentioned qualities of "demand" interventions can function as a framework for a mentalizing therapy process – a process, which may be considered beneficial for a wide range of patient groups. Due to the special challenges borderline patients may pose, keeping demand questions on the agenda, and not slipping on the subject, warrants intensive efforts on the therapist's behalf.

As for the interventional style of the PDG, possibly, neither the frequency of mentalizing-promoting interventions or intervention frequency in itself is high enough to actively lead patients in for longer streaks of mentalizing discourse, which may be a requisite for effective mentalizing work, as it may require a great deal of effort and motivation, and external structuring to achieve it (as seen in the MBT group).

Concluding remarks

In sum, our findings point to important differences between the groups. These differences coincide with central theoretical differences between the methods. Of course, the limited sample size pose limitations on generalizing the findings. Nevertheless, we believe that an analysis, such as ours, with some face validity can describe real differences between the methods which is relevant when considering therapeutic strategies. However, the differences between the groups may also be caused by other reasons, e.g., characteristics of the therapist's personality or style (the groups had different therapists), or that the current PDG was less representative than the MBT-group. A somewhat surprising observation was the highly supportive nature of the PDG, which was evident through the therapists' focus on seeking to help the patients via direct routes, for example, by focusing on the patients' progress and improvement, and showing support (Yalom & Leszcz, 2005). Also, abandoning the traditional challenging interpretative approach in favour of a more clarifying approach, reinforced this impression. Possibly, the analysis of the PDG may illustrate a common phenomenon, i.e. that therapies tend to drift towards supportive styles due to activation of attachment/care within the therapists in response to the despair of the patients (Karterud et al., 2016). In the latter case, this suggests that there is need for something extra to maintain a challenging demand attitude from the therapists, i.e. collegial support, supervision, a theory that justifies demand questions and explains the risk for a pseudomentalizing group discourse. In our study, the PDG had obviously drifted quite far from its group analytic ideals and origins. Accordingly, this study should be replicated before concluding its relevance for group analysis.

References

Antonsen, B. T., Klungsøyr, O., Johansen, M. S., Kemps, A., Pedersen, G., Hummelen, B., Urnes, U., Kvarstein, E., Karterud, S. & Wilberg, T. (2014). Step-down versus outpatient psychotherapeutic treatment for personality disorders: 6 years follow-up of the Ullevål Personality Project. *BMC Psychiatry*, 14: 119.

Bateman, A. & Fonagy, P. (1999). Effectiveness of partial hospitalization in the treatment pf borderline personality disorder: A randomized controlled trial. *American Journal of Psychiatry*, 156: 1563–1569.

Bateman, A. W. & Fonagy, P. (2004). *Psychotherapy for Borderline Personality Disorder. Mentalization-based Treatment*. Oxford: Oxford University Press.

Bateman, A. W. & Fonagy, P. (2006). *Mentalization Based Treatment for Borderline Personality Disorder: A Practical Guide*: Oxford: Oxford University Press.

Berghaus, A. & Potthoff, P. (2009). Gruppentherapie in der 'Postmoderne'—wie ändern sich Indikation und Technik? *Jahrbuch für Gruppenanalyse und ihre Anwendungen*, 14: 117–128.

Bion, W. R. (1970). *Attention and Interpretation*. London: Tavistock Publications.

Fonagy, P., Leigh, T., Steele, M., Steele, H., Kenedy, R., Mattoon, G., Target, M. & Gerber, A. (1996). The relation of attachment status, psychiatric classification, and responses to psychotherapy. *Journal of Consulting and Clinical Psychology*, 64: 22–31.

Fonagy, P., Target, M., Steele, H. & Steele, M. (1998). *Reflective Functioning Manual, Version 5.0, for Application to Adult Attachment Interviews*. London: University College London

Foulkes, S. H. (1964). *Therapeutic Group Analysis*. London: Karnac Books (reprinted 1984).

Glover, E. (1955). *The Technique of Psychoanalysis*. London: Bailliere Tindall and Co.

Gullestad, F., Wilberg, T., Klungsøyr, O., Urnes, Ø. & Karterud, S. (2012). Is treatment in a day hospital step-down program superior to outpatient individual psychotherapy for patients with personality disorders? – Results from a randomized clinical trial comparing different modalities. *Psychotherapy Research*, 22(4): 426–441.

Hesse, E. (2008). The adult attachment interview: Historical and current perspectives. In J. Cassidy & P. R. Shaver (Eds.), *Attachment Theory, Research and Clinical Application*. New York: Guilford Press

Karterud, S. (1999). *Gruppeanalyse og psykodynamisk gruppepsykoterapi*. Oslo: Pax.

Karterud, S. (2015). *Mentalization-based Group Therapy (MBT-G). A Theoretical, Clinical and Research Manual*. Oxford: Oxford University Press.

Karterud, S. (2018). A high-quality mentalization-based group therapy session. *Group Analysis*, 51(1): 18–43.

Karterud, S. & Bateman, A. (2011). *Manual for mentaliseringbasert psykoedukativ gruppeterapi (MBT-I)*. Oslo: Gyldendal Akademisk.

Karterud, S., Pedersen, G., Johansen, M., Wilberg, T., Davis, K. & Panksepp, J. (2016). Primary emotional traits in patients with personality disorders. *Personality and Mental Health*, 7(4): 1–13. DOI 10.1002/pmh.1345

Kernberg, O. F. (1984). *Severe Personality Disorders*. New Haven: Yale University Press.

Kohut, M. (1983). *The Restoration of the Self*. New York: International Universities Press.

Kvarstein, E., Pedersen, G., Urnes, Ø., Hummelen, B., Wilberg, T. & Karterud, S. (2014). Changing from a traditional psychodynamic treatment program to mentalization-based treatment for patients with borderline personality disorder. Does it make a difference? *Psychology and Psychotherapy: Theory, Research and Practice*, DOI: 10.1111/papt.12036

Lincoln, Y. & Guba, E. G. (1985). *Naturalistic Inquiry*. Newbury Park: Sage Publications.

Lorentzen, S. (2014). *Group Analytic Psychotherapy: Working with Affective, Anxiety and Personality Disorders*. UK: Routledge.

Merriam, S. B. (1988). *Case Study Research in Education: A Qualitative Approach*. San Francisco: Jossey–Bass.

Møller, C., Karlgren, L., Sandell, A., Falkenstrøm, F. & Philips, B. (2016). Mentalization-based therapy adherence and competence stimulates in-session mentalization in psychotherapy for borderline person personality disorder with co-morbid substance dependence. *Psychotherapy Research*, 27(6): 749–765.

Pedersen, S.-H., Lunn, S., Katznelson, H. & Poulsen, S. (2012). Reflective functioning in 70 patients suffering from bulimia nervosa. *European Eating Disorders Review*, 20: 303–310.

Potthoff, P. & Moini-Afchari, U. (2014). Mentalization-based treatment in groups – a paradigm shift or old wine in new skin? *Group Analysis*, 47(1): 3–16.

Rudolf, G. (2006). *Strukturbezogene Psychotherapie. Leitfaden zur psychodynamischen Therapie struktureller Störungen*. Stuttgart: Schattauer.

Schultz-Venrath, U. (2010). Editorial. *Psychotherapeut*, 55: 277–228.

Winnicott, D. W. (1971). *Playing and Reality*. London: Penguin Books.

Yalom, I. D. & Leszcz, M. (2005). *The Theory and Practice of Group Psychotherapy*. New York: Basic Books.

Zender, J. F. (1991). Projective identification in group psychotherapy. *Group Analysis*, 24(2): 117–129.

Zinkin, L. (1992). Borderline distortions of mirroring in the group. *Group Analysis*, 25(1): 27–31. doi: 10.1177/0533316492251005

Chapter 8

A high quality mentalization-based group therapy session

Sigmund Karterud

Abstract

A previous study of a MBT group displayed that the therapists failed to establish the group as a training ground for mentalizing. In this study we present a detailed and long transcript of a sequence in a successful MBT group. The therapists' interventions were rated according to the mentalization-based group therapy adherence and quality scale, performed by the Norwegian MBT Quality Laboratory. The therapists displayed a high adherence to the MBT-G manual, and the patients became collectively engaged in exploring and reflecting upon crucial borderline dynamics. The interventions that seemed most important for unfolding of the sequence are carefully spelled out. They have a metacognitive flavour but are elsewise simple and straight forward. There seems to be nothing essentially new in this MBT-G approach if one asks for specific ingredients. However, the therapeutic stance is consequently geared towards exploration of mental states, guided by a certain theory. One might say that it represents a more modern mixture of ingredients that are well known in different research and group therapy camps.

Introduction

In a previous article we (Indrehaug & Karterud, 2015) reported the results of a detailed qualitative study of a mentalization-based group (MBT-G) at a Norwegian Mental Health Centre. The results were disappointing. The group displayed most of the chaotic group transactions which MBT-G is supposed to counteract. We concluded that the therapists particularly failed in two important areas: 1) They had not gained and did not practice a firm authority as group leaders, and 2) they overplayed the principle of "not-knowing stance".

The above-mentioned study has left a void. The quantitative results of MBT as a conjoint individual-group therapy has been remarkably good (Kvarstein et al., 2014; Roussow & Fonagy, 2012; Bateman & Fonagy, 2009; Bales et al., 2012). However, there has not been published any qualitative study that has demonstrated how high quality MBT-G looks like. This paper aims to fill this void.

DOI: 10.4324/9781003625810-8

Material and methods

The group in this study belonged to the MBT program at Department of Personality Psychiatry, Oslo University Hospital. The video recording was done in January 2014. All patients and therapists gave their informed consent to participate in an exploratory study that aimed to compare MBT-G anno 2014 with a psychodynamic group therapy session *anno* 2006 (a historical record made for the Ullevål Personality Project (UPP; Antonsen et al., 2014). The group had been conducted according to MBT-G guidelines since 2008 and data from this group is part of the total data reported in Kvarstein et al. (2014). The findings from the comparative study are reported in a companion article (Kalleklev and Karterud, 2018). In this article we report on the MBT group only.

The six patients in the group were all female, mean age 30 years (range 23 – 40). Their personality problems were of the borderline type, while some also harboured avoidant features. Number of DSM-IV borderline criteria ranged from 4–8 (5 is diagnostic threshold and 9 is maximum). The patients also displayed a wide range of the typical symptom disorders which come with borderline PD, e.g., major depressive episodes, anxiety disorders, bulimia, substance use disorders. To be accepted for the MBT program their level of subjective distress should be high (with bouts of acting out) and their level of social functioning should be low (e.g., being unable to work or study for several years).

All patients had received 12 sessions of MBT psychoeducational group therapy during the first phase of their treatment (Karterud & Bateman, 2011). They had weekly individual MBT for about one year (thereafter more seldom) conjoint with MBT-G. Mean treatment time in this group was around 26 months. By the time of video recording, patient E was the most recent member (around six months in the group), while patient A was the most senior member (around 22 months in the group). The group lasted for 1,5 hours.

The group session was meticulously transcribed by a psychology student. All therapist interventions in the transcript (supported by the study of the video recording) were rated according to the mentalization-based group therapy adherence and quality scale (MBT-G-AQS). The rating was performed by the MBT quality laboratory at Oslo University Hospital. A recent reliability study of MBT-G-AQS has revealed high reliability, in the range of ICC-2: .80 -.90 (Folmo et al., 2017). The MBT-G-AQS is described in the manual by Karterud. It contains 19 items. Figure 8.1 displays the therapists′ adherence intervention profile. The therapists made in total 294 interventions. Of these 188 (64 % of total) were considered to comply with one or more of the MBT-G items. This is a high percentage compared to other (MBT-G) group sessions (Folmo et al., 2017). It is in itself an indicator of high MBT-G adherence. The intervention profile displays a rather balanced therapeutic style. The therapists used most of the 19 items, in particular the items on "mentalizing events in the group", "focus on emotions" and "working with the patient-therapist relationship". The overall rating for adherence was 7 and for

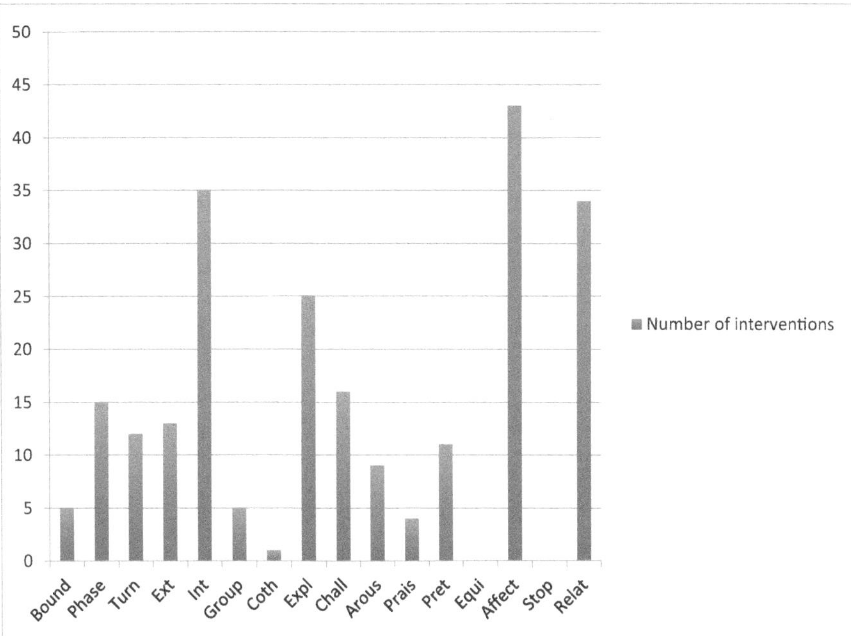

Figure 8.1 Bound = Managing group boundaries. Phase = Regulating group phases. Turn = Initiating and fulfilling turn-taking. Ext = Engaging members in mentalizing external events. Int = Identifying and mentalizing events in the group. Group = Stimulating discussions about group norms. Coth = Cooperation between co-therapists. Expl = Exploration, curiosity and not knowing stance. Chall = Challenging unwarranted believes. Arous = Regulating emotional arousal. Prais = Acknowledging good mentalization. Pret = Handling pretend mode. Equi = Handling psychic equivalence. Affect = focus on emotions. Stop = stop and rewind. Relat = Focus on the relationship between therapists and patients.

quality 6 (on a scale 1-7). Therapist 1 (T-1) was a qualified group analyst, well versed in MBT-G. Therapist 2 (T-2) was a psychiatric resident with no formal group therapy training.

The numbers in the preceding paragraph attest to a group session that might be said, according to established standards, to represent a high quality MBT-G session. How does that look like in more detail? In order to demonstrate that, we present most of the transcript of the longest "turn" in the group. All interventions are marked with notations like A-10 (adherence item 10), which denotes which item (of 19) the raters judged the intervention to belong to. Some interventions do not have any notation since they do not comply with any MBT item (e.g., "where did he live?").

The group started in a structured MBT way: All six patients were present. The therapists conveyed their thoughts about the group and all members from last session and asked for initiatives for this session. Two patients asked for attention. However, the therapists explained that they also would like to hear something from patient L, since she had been mentioned only briefly the last sessions and since there was a long time since she had entered the group stage. The reader should be informed that L at this point had recovered very much from the turbulent and chaotic lifestyle she exhibited at the beginning of treatment. However, lately she had been a rather passive member of the group. She had been in treatment for around 20 months.

The opening phase of the group lasted for around 7 minutes. Thereafter comes this sequence with L which lasted for around 40 minutes. It was followed by a sequence with patient A (centring on her recovery process and termination) and a sequence with patient B (centring on her memory deficits, including not remembering what happens in the group).

Results

The sequence with patient L, after seven minutes:

"T2: Well, where should we begin, should we start with … (looks around) … would you (looks at patient L) start, perhaps? (A-3)

L: (Smiles) Honestly, I have no idea of anything to say. I don't have a clue. There is nothing I have been thinking on … or any event, or something which I … I have no idea of what to talk about … (laughs) to be totally honest.

T2: I … believe it was kind of like this also last time we … (A-4)

L: No … yes, perhaps it was… but there surfaced something, nevertheless. Was it that session you had in mind?

T2: Mm

L: Eh … yes, it was. But that time I had something in mind although I pretended I had not, but I haven't that now … (laughter). I promise … it's true. It's true … no, there isn't that much … time is consumed by … I'm waiting for moving out, so the situation at home is quite strange … and in a way … energy is sucked by those thoughts, so I haven't much else in a way … am in a kind of middle phase. So … yes …

T2: Thoughts and energy are preoccupied …?

L: It's hard to live at home … when you are to be separated and … the situation is strange … and it's very hard for both parties, and in a way … how should you relate to each other and … well it goes very well, but in a way … both of us know that it is only a waiting period … so it's a kind of …

T2: Does he have bouts of rage? Or is he more steady…?(A-17, 11)

L: No, not particularly … he is like he uses to be, in a way, not on to me … well not very much.

T2: No.

L: He did not react in the way I feared … he hasn't done that…

T2: So, he did agree with you?

T1: But, when you explain it in this way, it seems like it will depend on us, eh … eh … well, what do we think around the fact that you have nothing particular to talk about? Then we might think, and I think like this, that two issues pop up: No, perhaps you do not have anything to talk about because everything is OK … but if so… should we then talk about termination? Because, if everything is OK, then there is no reason to come to the group. Because this is therapy. Or do you say that you don't have anything … because that's the very problem which should be addressed? (A-19, 11)

L: Yes …

T1: So, what might it be?

L: I have to say …

T1: How should we relate to … how should we understand this and relate to it? (A-19, 11)

L: I'll try to remember what I discussed with my individual therapist last session … because we discussed something around what I should work with. Because we have talked about termination this autumn …

T1: Or perhaps you should terminate earlier? (A-13)

L: Or … or it … (laughs) … don't know really, because I haven't talked about it, but I would very much like to have … in any case, a tiny contact here since … my life situation will be quite different and I don't know how I will react, in a way, and such things, so I wouldn't like to somehow: "OK, now we terminate, because things for the future are settled". But now I try to remember what my therapist and I talked about, what I should … yes, no, it concerned that I need to work on the issue of being more outspoken. To voice my feelings and tell … it mostly concerns when others are talking. Because I often just sit there, and I feel sort of things, but I do not bother to tell it … or I do not tell it … or … yes, I might be annoyed, or I might be … yes … such things. Eh, that was the kind of things I should … try out, get some training. I do not quite remember what …

Patient N: Can I ask you … (to L)? Is it like that … in a way … when someone else talks about something, … and then … does it evoke feelings in … own feelings in you? Or is it more like that you might be annoyed because you think they are sulking, or you think that they don't do what they should … or?

T2: Here in the group? (A-5)

L: I often think that people are just sulking, but often it concerns other things. Maybe it concerns … Very often I get irritated when there might be other kind of feelings that … there are other reasons for my emotions … but quite often … the first thing that comes is annoyance. And then … but that's what I have neglected … then I, since I get so annoyed, … should try to find out what's behind that emotion. Because … usually it's not the case that what the person says is that stupid. Often it is other things. Well … I believe so … yes.

Patient E: It's important to receive negative comments too.

L: Yes …

E: Because … if I say something, it might be productive, in a way, to receive … negative feedback

L: Yes …

E: Because then … it might help me to find out more about myself. It isn't such that …

T1: Wow, that was … (laughs)

E: Yes, because this is not a support group, is it?

T1: No, I agree. This is not a support group (group laughter). This is … an active work group. (A-7)

E: Yes

T1: So, it was only a bit surprising to … to hear that … I found those comments from your side positive. Kind of "yes, we are here in order to work" and that includes critical feedback. (A-14)

E: People must not be afraid of …

T2: Did you believe she had … since you said what you said? Did you believe … (A-11)

E: No, but if there is something I have said … and if she has thought … then it is important to receive that feedback

T2: Do you wonder if, actually … if L has (L interrupts) (A-11)

L: I believe it is you, therapist T2, that wonders (looks at T2 and laughs)

E: No (laughs)

T2: No, but you may ask (A-5)

E: No, but … yes if I say something, indeed I should receive feedback

L: (nods) Yes, it's good to know … but it wasn't …

Patient N: I agree.

L: You too? (looks at N)

N: I don't say that I will take it nicely (group laughter), but surely, I would learn something.

L: But it often turns out that I … often I do not … I don't say anything because I know … or I believe … I don't know exactly what it is. Sometimes it isn't … it isn't certain that it serves any purpose, because my … in a way, my harsh way to give feedback, perhaps is due to other things … so that … I'm not sure if it is to any help for that other person, because it concerns other feelings inside me, which is … which I have not sorted out … or I don't know … in a way … anger and annoyance come very fast … and those feelings are linked to all feelings.

N: Yes, but then we get to know it … and we might work on it.

E: Yes.

T2: Yes, because I can … I'm sitting here trying to remember … have you ever been openly angry here? (A-5, 17)

L: No.

T2: After I joined the group? (A-5)

L: No, I don´t believe so.

N: You were often angry with Mary (previous therapist in the group)

L: (laughs) She … yes, perhaps I was.

T2: Was it visible? (A-17)

N: You stopped Mary if she said anything stupid or … if you did not understand what she said and things like that. You often did that. But it was OK.

Patient P: Quite a few of us thought that … (is interrupted by N)

N: It was like … we had many of the same feelings, but you were good at speaking out.

L: Ah, I don't remember that.

N: It was fine.

T1: Mm … OK, so there is something here, after all? (A-13, 15)

L: Yes … and it isn't that I in some way … eh … deny that I do it. Because I do, but I have great difficulties in finding out these things, so in a way you are right … when I say that there isn't anything … it need not be anything in particular, but there are themes I should work with, like those I have mentioned.

T1: Mm

L: Like … because I have wondered, I've thought a lot about … that … there is something that I asked for when I started here, in treatment, that I wanted to get more in touch with my emotions and be more confident with them. And … eh … then I have in a way discovered … or got to know it in a way … that annoyance is a feeling that takes precedence to all other feelings. I do not feel sorrow, I get annoyed … I do not get such … I get irritated. And then it is basically something else.

T1: Possibly. (A-15)

L: And it might … yes, often it might be … and sometimes I'm just annoyed and … it might be. But … eh … I know for example that often … often in therapy settings, somebody says something, for example a psychologist who says something which possibly hits the target, I become incredibly angry. And then I don't manage … or I become incredible irritated and then … Previously I just got irritated and believed I hated that person and that there were quite other reasons, but lately I have understood that, the reaction now use to come in the aftermath when I reflect upon it that "Ah, there was something in what she said that made me … it was … it was unpleasant", but previously I have thought that I just don't like that person, and I have searched for reasons to justify that I do not like her, because she did such and such, but now I have understood that I have been unjust, that it is not always what I believed it to be. When somebody evokes something unpleasant in me …

T1: Well, but how should we handle this since you have got accustomed to a passive role? (A-19, 5)

L: Well, it's something that I must do myself … I can … and you can help … yes, that was what I talked to my therapist about, that I … that I, in a way, should speak out that I had problems with these things … and that I … in a way should become more conscious at … and you would be too. And that we in a way should try to … yes … to do something with it. That was what she said, I believe.

T1: But how should we … how should we handle this? It is … (A-19, 5)

L: I'll have to do the most myself, really.

T1: So, it is … well, firstly it requires …

L: Yes, I believe she said that one should check in with, or … but then I risk "I cannot be so preoccupied with myself the whole time», but … that you can ask me … I don't know. You can ask me when I ... I don't know.

N: But it will be easier … like now, when everybody is aware of it, in a way …

L: Yes.

N: and then they know that … and if everybody agrees … and you know that it is accepted for you to intrude if you in a way … when you.

L: Yes, that might be … perhaps it will be more easy … we will see … yes

T1: Mm … OK … OK. But to get straight to the matter. When was the last time you were irritated here in the group? (A-5, 13, 17)

L: I get annoyed every time.

Group laughter

T1: Yes, OK, so last time … what and who annoyed you? (A-5, 17)

L: Ah … I remember poorly what was up last time and what … what did we talk about? It was your (looks at patient E) father and things … That did not annoy me. And then it was your (looks at patient N) … No, I was not that annoyed last time actually, because it was … eh … you talked about what had happened. But I got irritated the session before that.

T1: OK.

L: Eh … then I got irritated … eh … when it was …

T1: At whom? (A-5)

L: At many.

T1: Yes.

Group laughter

L: Eh … I got irritated at you. (points at T1)

T1: Yes, OK. (A-19)

L: Because you stressed … it was when … when we had that issue about the absences of patient N.

T1: Yes.

L: Then I got … but there are different kinds of annoyances.

T1: Yes.

L: But then I got irritated, actually. And it was … it wasn't anything more behind it …

T1: No

L: It was because I thought she was hanging somehow in very thin air and she got bewildered since she did not receive any feedback … but she was forced to the wall and it was incredible detailed … and it lasted … and often I can become irritated when I feel that things are damned stretched, and that you … eh … I don't know. I do not always understand what you are up to, but sometimes I understand that I also might be wrong. Because suddenly you have arrived at something, but I often believe … when you talk (looks at T1) … when you talk, because you have such a calm voice and when … and sometimes I slip out a bit (laughter) when you become … tell kind of things. It's not that I … and sometimes I can … that is very … it's very awkward to say, but … when someone says … and it is really bad of me …

N: Come on!

L: Yes, … no, when someone says like … and you said that you (points at E) in a way didn't get up in the morning … and you (points at N) said you were so tired. I cannot … I have hard to … I understand that you are not sitting there lying, but I do not manage to mobilize that much sympathy with you. I find it difficult. I've turned like "hell, just do what you should do", that's one side of me, but another side is different because I know that you (looks at N) do not just sit there and pretend that you cannot do anything. I don't know … I believe it comes from … it has to come from somewhere. It comes from home, from all the sulking. My mother was like "I cannot this, couldn't that, couldn't cope», so I believe I have a very low threshold for such kind of things. Often when I get irritated on how people behave, it's because it reminds me of something. E.g., I had this therapist that reminded me about my mother. It was the worst thing I ever encountered (laughter). It didn't go well.

T1: No …

L: So, it is …

T1: So, it is … yes. T2 does not remind you of your mother? (A-19)

L: No.

T1: Good to hear. (A-19)

L: Not you either. (laughter)
T1: No, not I either. (laughs). (A-19)
L: But (looks at N), did you feel lousy when I said it?
N: Mm…mm..
L: Yes, you did … and then I get …
N: No, but no, I think … I think that it is quite OK that you say so, but of course it evokes feelings in me, because I eh … get guilt feelings when I don't manage to do things.
L: Yes, and that's why I have thought that I really should not say it, because … I do not believe that you …
N: Well, yes … it's quite OK that you say it, because …
L: Yes, but I …
N: Yes, but these … well, in a way it's like the way you express it. In a way it is … eh …well it is thoughts that pop up in all kind of people around.
L: Yes.
N: When you have to withdraw from things because you are ill or tired or kind of things. Then it's such that I …
L: Yes, but it's like … (N disrupts)
N: I must cope with that … that other people harbour such opinions.
L: Yes, but I will not that you should believe, in a way … because, in a way it's divided in two. I see … because I do not believe that you are lying.
N: No, no
L: But at the same time, I've difficulties with understanding …
N: No, I do not get sad because you say so. But it evokes feelings, it does. But I don't get … it's not like I'm getting angry with you, or …
L: But I get a bit … like … annoyed at myself or a bit like … at myself sometimes because I …
N: But that doesn't make me afraid. I don't think it's … I don't think it's wrong by you to say so.
L: No.
N: When you … when you get those feelings, like «OK, yes … but what's behind these things? Why? …", you should address it.
L: Yes … yes.
N: So, in a way … it's OK that you have this opinion. It's …
T1: Mm … yes, but it clearly seems to be the case that this (points at L) hasn't been easy for you. (A-5, 17)
L: I'm stressed as hell.
T1: Yes, so these things were not easy to express. Clearly it evoked … (A-5, 17)
L: Oh yea, God.
T1: And what is it … when it …(A-5, 11)
L: No, I believe I will undo it. It hurts.
Several: Laughter

T1: Yes, what … what is going on inside you? Is it that …(A-5, 17)

L: That she (N) … that I have hurt her.

T1: That you have done her harm? Yes? (A-17)

L: Oh … yes.

T1: Well … the way I look upon it, I don't know how you other here look upon it, but I think that, yes, perhaps you evoked some pain, but … but … to evoke some pain and frustrate other people, might be one should do that now and then. It wasn't … it wasn't too bad, you (to patient N) didn't collapse, it seemed like you could take it. (A-5, 17)

T2: What do you think about this (to the group members)? (A-5)

L: Well, one thing which I know is a problem for me, that's a feeling that I should … that whole my life I have … if I could choose, I would prefer to do harm to myself before others. I prefer to … eh … to say that things are OK when they are not OK, to protect another … and I can say things, and do things, which I dislike, to protect other people. It's very pervasive, and this is something that I would like to work on.

T1: Mm … mm … yes, you (to T2) asked how people reacted at … (A-9)

T2: Yes, how are your thoughts about being that open? (A-8)

E: I think it's perfectly OK.

T2: Yes, you said so some minutes ago

E: Yes, but eh … like you said … I don't understand why people don't just stand up and do it. It's exactly the same thoughts that I have been saying to myself. So … it's nothing new to me.

T1: But what about the fact that N felt this as very unpleasant? (A-5, 17)

E: Yes, I see that. But it was not that unpleasant. She expressed herself in a very fine way.

N: Yes, and it is not the case that I would have it undone

T2: Yes, because for you … in a way … these are things about yourself which you know about (looks at N) (A-11)

N: Well … I mean, it's … of course I too get angry with myself. Why don't I succeed? Why can't I just do it? Even … those eating problems … I cannot do so much with them, but of course … I know there are situations where I in a way … I do not quite understand why I don't manage … and I should work on that … and sometimes I'm frustrated with myself because I feel I should have managed … really … I could have done it. In other occasions I might feel the same although it's beyond my capabilities. You see … it's difficult, but that people think like that … I'm having the same thoughts myself, everybody has, about other people. I believe most of us have, like «just pull yourself together», even if I hate to hear it, I think … I think that … most people think like that about others.

T1: What kind of thoughts did you (to patient S) have? (A-5)

S: Eh … I get … annoyed when I hear «pull yourself together», but I too have such thoughts about others. I get pissed off when people just sit there and behave helpless.

T2: Eh … yes, wait … just stop a second. You get annoyed when people say, "pull yourself together". So you got annoyed with patient L when she … (A-5, 17)

S: A bit. I've heard it damned lot of times myself … "pull yourself together"

T2: Ok, so it might resonate with other experiences you have, or?

S: Oh … yes. I don't know, I'm very divided. Eh … I think like that about my mother because she is so damned helpless, and I think "God … shape up! You are so pitiful!", and then I get annoyed. But I'm thinking that I'm exactly like that myself, and I hate to hear it from others. Because it is not easy to pull oneself together.

A short sequence with patient S is deleted because of space limitation.

N: I understood … you really found good words for what I'm feeling … and that is such a divided feeling … that in a way … one hates to hear it, because … at least me, I've heard it in so many situations when I actually was so ill that I did not have any choice. And that's why it might sound very unjust. But of course, I understand that, in a way … there's nobody who really understand the state of other people, and I understand that from the outside it might … that people might think. And sometimes it might well be justified.

L: For me it's also a kind of divided thing, because I have my thoughts while I at the same time I understand there is something else. But anyhow, this irritation pops up, even if one knows … it's like …

S: If you had just said "Pull yourself together" and that's it … full stop … haven't said anything more, then I would have become furious.

L: Yes, but I didn't mean it like that: "Patient N, pull yourself together!" It was rather a way of … that I have harboured such thoughts now and then. And not only … well, I think like that about many people, and I get kind of bad conscience because I think such thoughts.

N: Yes, I've thought like that many times about people here.

L: You think, and then you get like … you feel very little empathic afterwards, but it's like … it's those emotions … they come anyhow, in a way.

T1: Patient P, where are you in all this? (A-4)

There follows a short sequence where patient P says she "agrees with everybody" (with humour), that she is reluctant to grab more attention, but that she had been open with her feelings toward the "stern eyes" of T1, and that it was OK to have said that.

T1: But anyhow, for you (looks at L) it is an important theme that you get … you get some unpleasant feelings when you believe you have hurt someone or been a burden to somebody. (A-17, 7)

L: Mm … yes, but I have to say one thing, that … that in real life I'm very, very careful. But here, actually it turned out to be fine. Because it is something which has scared me more than anything else … it's like, in a way … my pattern is that I have thought in the aftermath "What's going to happen now?" It's like … it feels like the world is falling apart.

T2: Also here?

L: Yes, if I do something … yes, not now … not now. This time it actually went fine. But … hurting others … that … I don't know what I believe …

T2: Have you tried? Is it possible to … ask … how?

L: Yes, one should. But, in a way … I don't dare to say such … usually out there, but now …

T1: Mm … seems like a pattern for you.

L: Yes, yes.

T1: Like a personality trait?

L: Yes.

T1: Which obviously must be burdensome.

L: Yes, and I needed it in my earlier life, but I don't need to have it any longer.

T1: No … Do you have … do you know … why you have become this way? (A-11)

L: Eh … it's from early years. It was so stormy … so incredibly much quarrelling and shouting and everything, so I believe I just adopted a kind of mediator role, in a way and I had … I felt a strong responsibility for everybody. So, I believe that I feel, in a way, a strong responsibility for people I don't know also. Because I do not dare to hurt even people I do not know. I guess I feel some responsibility. I know … well, I don't know really … it's complex, may be. But it is this … it's this case that I cannot stand that distress. I … well, I cannot cope with those unpleasant feelings. I will rather in a way … take the blame on me, make them angry with me or being pissed off because of me. Then I will get the pain.

T1: And the pain … and you … (A-17)

L: It's so painful that I don't know what I shall …

T1: Well … and then you …? What's the name of the pain? (A-17)

L: Eh … I don't know, but it is … name? But it's very … eh … it's a kind of pain that … Now I must learn to feel it and … to realize that the world does not succumb when I'm in pain, but previously it was like … I didn't let it … once it was there, I had to do something, in a way, to let off steam or to … often when I said something I really meant, I would often undo it, or deny it or withdraw it, and try to clean up. And I would stay with people I basically didn't want to hang around with. It's been like that, turning towards myself rather than onto others.

T1: Yes … do you other (in the group) have any opinion on the name of this pain? (A-4, 17)

E: Bad conscience.

T1: You think it might be bad conscience?

E: Which likely comes too easy.

L: Yes, I have.

T1: Yes, it is …?

L: Yes, I've bad conscience for everything. For things that have no connection to my own faults. Everything, in a way.

T2: What's your thoughts about this (looks at patient A)? (A-4)

A: Hm?

T2: What're your thoughts about this feeling? (A-11, 17)

A: I don't know … I've forgotten that feeling. I don't have this feeling, so I don't know what it means.

T2: Does that mean that if you confront somebody, about something, if you get annoyed or you express your opinion, are you through with it? (A-17)

A: Yes, quite through.

T1: But what if you have hurt somebody? (A-12)

A: I don't believe I do hurt anybody.

T1: No, never? (A-12)

A: Well, it might be, but … no, I have a maxim that I should be accountable for everything I say, but I cannot be responsible for how other reacts.

T2: My first thought was that «well, that might be a good rule of life», but then I thought "don't you ever reflect upon the effects of your actions? Do you try to avoid them?" Is that what you mean? (A-15, 19)

N: I believe it's a bit avoidance of responsibility.

A: No, I don't agree. It's the way I said it … I can face up to it. If I say something which make people feel … that I'm evil, then they have to tell me why they react in this way, and then I might explain myself. It's communication.

T1: Mm … OK. You have never experienced bad conscience? (A-17)

A: I had much of it previously, but I have got rid of it. If I should go around with bad conscience for everything I say and do, and avoid this and that, then …

T1: I don't say that … that you should. I just wonder how … but when you say that you have difficulties with identifying that feeling …(A-12, 15, 17)

A: Yes, because these days I do not go around thinking that I have or that I should have bad conscience.

T1: Yes, because now we have said in a way that this is the nature of your feelings (nods at patient L): Bad conscience. (A-17)

L: Yes, it's kind of …

T1: And you (looks at E) … you nodded.

L: Yes, it's in a way … yes, I have that too … very much bad conscience, but … I guess it's kind of mixture … I have very bad conscience eh … generally, but eh …it surely is, but eh … I cannot stand that other people are in pain, and certainly not if it is because of me. Then I have to do something. I turn … I turned … and I know that it comes from childhood, from mama, because she cried all the time, and I had to, I had to fix or do and do something, but don't want to have it like that now.

T1: No.

L: It's not good for me.

T1: Yes, but it is deeply anchored. (A-17)

L: Yes, but I'm thinking … well, I think in a way … if one should be serious, I believe I didn't want to stay in any of the relationships … perhaps one … perhaps it it's been one relationship in my life that I really wanted. So it's in a way … if I really think to the bottom of things, I've never realized … or, if somebody liked me or did care for me, I did it for their sake.

T1: Yes, you did things for others.

L: Yes, I do … and I may like people too. But I'm too … I'm too adaptable. I'm so adaptable that I don't know what's left of me, in a way. And what defines my own self. I believe … when I'm together with someone, that I like, or prefer this or that, while when I'm with someone else, I …
(in the following sequence she speaks about the man she loved, how he died, about her strivings to get out of her current relationship and the temptations to remain and get seduced by phrases like "but I love you", etc.) After around 45 minutes:

T1: OK … seems to be time to proceed … If we look back, we took the initiative to hook you in. (A-2)

L: Yes.

T1: How was it for you to be hooked in that manner? (A-2, 19)

L: It was fine. Good. Yes …

T1: Mm … so next time you'll hook on more by yourself? (A-2)

L: Yes, I'll try, I'll try. I believe it then will be easier, because in a way I have …

T1: Mm … yes … OK"

The session proceeds with one sequence with A as the protagonist (around her termination and what has been most helpful during the treatment) and, thereafter, a sequence with S (around her memory problems, focused on how they manifest themselves in the group).

Discussion

We have presented a detailed verbatim account of what happened in the dominant sequence of a mentalization-based group session in a well-established MBT program which is known to have very good treatment results (Kvarstein et al., 2014). Patients in this program, even they are often labelled "difficult to treat" patients (Roth, Stone, & Kibel, 1990), benefit from effect sizes (range 1.4 – 1.7) that are around twice as large as what is ordinarily regarded as "good" in psychotherapy (Wampold, 2001). The session was not chosen because we knew on beforehand that it was exceptionally good or something like that. However, the therapists knew that the session was recorded for research purposes. That may have influenced their performance. However, there are reasons to believe that this session was fairly representative for the group in question. The ratings displayed a very high adherence to the MBT-G manual. By the verbatim account we have presented, the reader should get a good "feel" of the discourse style, what MBT-G looks or sounds like, and might compare it to other modes of group psychotherapy. In the following we will highlight some crucial features.

The opening phase is short, according to the manual, and sort of "business as usual" (Karterud, 2015). The members of the group are well versed with the structural characteristics of MBT-G. However, it seems to come as a surprise (for patient L, not for the other patients) when the therapists suggest that L should start. L starts in a non-mentalizing mode. She's empty. There is nothing there to talk about, nothing which evokes her curiosity. It might be OK to be in a non-mentalizing mode in other circumstances, but not in psychotherapy. In this case, T2 tries to be helpful by asking about any problems in her current relationship. We note that this intervention fails. It asks about some mental content in a self-state characterized by non-mentalizing. T1 adopts quite a different perspective. It's a meta-perspective on the situation here and now, directed at L, but simultaneous and explicitly to the group as a whole, and the intervention calls for mentalizing and metacognition (Main, 1991; Dimaggio & Lysaker, 2015): *"What do we think about this and how should we relate to our thoughts?"* This intervention is the major turning point. From then on L tries to work and her mentalizing capacity gradually recovers and becomes used for exploration of quite intriguing mental phenomena. She starts by trying to remember the words of her individual therapist. She enters a track of interpersonal transactions, about suppressing feelings in the here and now. The discourse is still somewhat abstract or generalized, until T1 says: *"OK, but to go straight to the matter. When were you irritated last time in this group?"* This intervention is very simple and straight forward. It complies with the overall aim of MBT-G: using the group as a training ground for mentalizing. It asks for an "event" which everybody in the group has witnessed, which is interpersonal and loaded with feelings. Not surprisingly, it raises the "temperature". Group members get involved with a current group theme, e.g., how frank and open should one be about own thoughts and feelings. L is the most restricted one, while the others call for more "enabling group solutions", to use the phrase of Dorothy Withaker (1981). By this exchange L's thwarted interpersonal pattern becomes visible in the here and now. If the reader goes back to the transcript, he/she will note that the therapists are not particular active or dominant through this sequence. This is not any kind of "individual therapy in group" with the other group members as onlookers. It's definitely "psychotherapy through the group process". Fellow patients spontaneously join the discussion and those that are more hesitant are asked by the therapists. All present group members participate. They comment upon L's dilemmas and reveal some personal comments that resonate with the current theme. However, nobody "steals" the attention. The attention is soon back to L who is the defined protagonist and who "owns" the sequence. The group members struggle with the difficult theme of how to cope with "bad" aspects (hostile thoughts) of themselves. It's noteworthy that this theme does not evoke splitting (which often will be the case with such patients). The "solution" is rather to accept and own "bad me" and try to find an acceptable outlet for it. This is most difficult for patient L since it evokes such painful feelings.

The next crucial intervention is when *T1 asks for a name for these feelings*. This is a "classical" MBT intervention. The therapist resists the temptation to come with an interpretation or doing the mentalizing job himself. By then everybody in the group has heard of some "painful feelings", but less about the nature or name of these feelings. Also, this time the intervention is very simple and straightforward. L has difficulties with labelling the feelings, while E quickly defines them as "bad conscience". This label is used for some time, although L describes the feelings as mixed and complex. T1 acknowledge this mixed nature and his next intervention spurs L into a more complex exploration of her difficulties with other people, describing her boundary problems, how the feelings of others tend to become her feelings. By her own words she describes what we usually define as projective identification. She then elaborates on her interpersonal subjugation and how that affects her identity. *The classical borderline pathology is clearly spelled out: The childhood family turmoil, the insecure attachment pattern, the effort to "save" other significant persons at the expense of sound emotion regulation for her own sake and at the expense of identity disturbance, resulting in destructive interpersonal relations in adult life. She ends up by describing how this pattern risks undermining her efforts to break out of her current destructive relationship.*

This long story was not delivered in any readymade pseudomentalizing, manner. At least parts of it were gained through a struggle here and now in the group since her pattern also materialized here and now and required the help of others, e.g., the therapists and fellow group members, to be seen and to be verbalized and reflected upon. By default, L would prefer to be a passive defiant group member (at the risk of being exploited once more). During this session she moved from a non-mentalizing mode to a fairly high reflective functioning (around 5-7 on the RF scale, Fonagy, Target, Steele, & Steele, 1998).

In summary, the crucial interventions were 1) the initial one that called for mentalizing and metacognition, 2) the one that asked for the here and now group example, and 3) the one that asked for the name of the feelings ("mentalizing affects"). All these interventions were formulated in a manner that also invited the other group members to partake, and they took the opportunity.

I believe that group therapists from different camps would agree with many of the considerations above and conclude that this is a piece of good therapeutic work with difficult to treat patients. The style might possibly appeal more to therapist of (American) psychodynamic group orientation (Rutan, Stone, & Shay, 2007), and possibly the most to interpersonal colleagues (Yalom & Leszcz, 2005; Marsiali & Munroe-Blum, 1994). The direct and challenging approach towards singular patients and the way of devoting so much time and attention to that patient, may seem alien for group analysts. On the other hand, they may appreciate the way the therapists work through the group (Pines, 1990). It is noteworthy that the therapists´ stance is consequently geared towards exploration of mental states. This is possibly the hallmark of the approach: That the therapists engage the other group members in exploring mental states rather than explaining or interpreting them.

Potthoff and Moini-Afchari (2014) discuss if MBT represents a paradigmatic shift or if it really offers anything essential new. Paradigmatic shifts in the strong sense of the word do not occur, or do so extremely seldom, in the social sciences. And it's hard to detect any "essential new" elements when we scrutinize the transcript above. The elements, i.e. the therapist interventions, are well known for experienced group therapists. However, we might introduce some new metaphors: The ingredients are well known, but the dish is somewhat different. And that's because the recipe (the manual) is different. And the manual is different because it integrates new basic research findings, e.g., on evolution (Panksepp & Biver, 2012), Theory of Mind experiments (Call & Tomasello, 2008) primary emotions (Karterud et al., 2016), attachment, implicit and explicit mentalizing (Fonagy, Bateman, & Bateman, 2011), cognition and metacognition (Tomasello, 2014), self-development (Sharp, Fonagy, & Goodyer, 2008; Bogdan, 2010), with personality and intersubjective deficits (Karterud, Wilberg, & Urnes, 2017), and psychotherapy effects (Kvarstein et al., 2014), in a different way than other textbooks/manuals. One might label it more "modern". In a companion article we will discuss how this approach is different and similar to group analytic oriented psychotherapy.

References

Antonsen, B. T., Klungsøyr, O., Kamp, A., Hummelen, B., Johansen, M. S., Pedersen, G., Urnes, Ø., Kvarstein, E. H., Karterud, S. & Wilberg, T. (2014). Step-down versus outpatient psychotherapeutic treatment for personality disorders: 6 years follow-up of the Ullevål personality project. *BMC Psychiatry,* 14(119). doi: 10.1186/1471-244X-14-119

Bales, D., van Beek, N., Smits, M., Willemsen, S., Bussbach, J. J. V., Verheul, R. & Andrea, H. (2012). Treatment outcome of 18-month, day hospital mentalization-based treatment

(MBT) in patients with severe borderline personality disorder in the Netherlands. *Journal of Personality Disorders*, 26(4): 568–582.

Bateman, A. & Fonagy, P. (2009). Randomized controlled trial of outpatient mentalization-based treatment versus structured clinical management for borderline personality disorder. *American Journal of Psychiatry*, 166: 1355–1364.

Bogdan, R. J. (2010). *Our Own Minds. Sociocultural Grounds for Self-consciousness.* London: The MIT Press.

Call, J. & Tomasello, M. (2008). Does the chimpanzee have a theory of mind: 30 years later. *Trends in Cognitive Science*, 12: 87–92.

Dimaggio, G. & Lysaker, P. H. (2015). Metacognition and mentalizing in the psychotherapy of patients with psychosis and personality disorders. *Journal of Clinical Psychology*, 71(2): 117–124.

Folmo, E., Karterud, S., Bremer, K., Walter, K. L., Kvarstein, E. & Pedersen, G. A. F. (2017). The design of the MBT-G adherence and quality scale. *Scandinavian Journal of Psychology*, 58: 341–349.

Fonagy, P., Bateman, A. & Bateman A (2011). The widening scope of mentalizing: A discussion. *Psychology and Psychotherapy: Theory, Research and Practice*, 84, 98–110.

Fonagy, P., Target, M., Steele, H. & Steele, M. (1998). *Reflective-Functioning Manual, Version 5, for Application to Adult Attachment Interviews*. University College London, unpublished manuscript.

Indrehaug, T. S. & Karterud, S. (2015). A qualitative study of a mentalization-based group for borderline patients. *Group Analysis*, 48(2): 150–163.

Kalleklev, J. & Karterud, S. (2018). A comparative study of mentalization-based versus psychodynamic group therapy. *Group Analysis*, 51(1): 44–60.

Karterud, S. & Bateman, A. (2011). *Manual for mentaliseringbasert psykoedukativ gruppeterapi (MBT-I). (A Manual for mentalization-based psychoeducative group therapy.).* Oslo: Gyldenal Akademisk.

Karterud, S. (2015). *Mentalization-based Group Therapy (MBT-G): A Theoretical, Clinical and Research Manual.* London: Oxford University Press.

Karterud, S., Wilberg, T. & Urnes, Ø. (2017). *Personlighetspsykiatri* ("Personality Psychiatry"). Oslo: Gyldendal Akademisk.

Karterud, S., Pedersen, G., Johansen, M., Wilberg, T., Davis, K. & Panksepp, J. (2016). Primary emotional traits in patients with personality disorders. *Journal of Personality and Mental Health*, 1–13. DOI 10.1002/pmh.1345

Kvarstein, E., Pedersen, G., Urnes, Ø., Hummelen, B., Wilberg, T. & Karterud, S. (2014). Changing from a traditional psychodynamic treatment program to mentalization-based treatment for patients with borderline personality disorder. Does it make a difference? *Psychology and Psychotherapy: Theory, Research and Practice*, 88(1): 71–86. DOI: 10.1111/papr.12036

Main, M. (1991). Metacognitive knowledge, metacognitive monitoring and singular (coherent) vs. multiple (incoherent) model of attachment: Findings and direction for future research. In C. M. Parkes, I. Stephenson-Hinde, & P. Marris (Eds.), *Attachment Across the Life Cycle* (pp. 127–159). London: Routledge Press.

Marsiali, E. & Munroe-Blum, H. (1994). *Interpersonal Group Psychotherapy for Borderline Personality Disorder.* New York: Basic Books.

Panksepp, J. & Biven, L. (2012). *The Archeology of Mind. Neuroevolutionary Origins of Human Emotions.* New York: W.W. Norton & company.

Potthoff, P. & Moini-Afchari, U. (2014). Mentalization-based treatment in groups – a paradigm shift or old wine in new skin? *Group Analysis,* 47(1): 3–16.

Pines, M. (1990). Group analytic psychotherapy and the borderline patient. In B. E. Roth, W. N. Stone, & H. D. Kibel (Eds.), *The Difficult Patient in Group*. Madison: International Universities Press.

Rossouw, T. & Fonagy, P. (2012). Mentalization-based treatment for self-harm in adolescents: A randomized controlled trial. *Journal of the American Academy of Child & Adolescent Psychiatry*, 51(12): 1304–1313.

Roth, B. E., Stone, W. N. & Kibel, H. D. (Eds.) (1990). *The Difficult Patient in Group.* Madison: International Universities Press.

Rutan, S. C., Stone, W. N. & Shay, J. J. (2007). *Psychodynamic Group Psychotherapy*. New York: The Guilford Press.

Sharp, C., Fonagy, P. & Goodyer, I. (Eds.) (2008). *Social Cognition and Developmental Psychopathology.* Oxford: Oxford University Press.

Tomasello, M. (2014). *A Natural History of Human Thinking.* London: Harvard University Press.

Yalom, I. D. & Leszcz, M. (2005). *The Theory and Practice of Group Psychotherapy.* New York: Basic Books.

Wampold, B. E. (2001). *The Great Psychotherapy Debate: Model, Methods and Findings.* Mahwah: Lawrence Erlbaum Associates.

Whitaker, D. S. (1981). A nuclear conflict and group focal conflict model for integrating individual and group-level phenomena in psychotherapy groups. In M. Pines & L. Rafaelsen (Eds.), *The Individual and the Group: Boundaries and Interrelations in Theory and Practice.* New York: Plenum Press.

Chapter 9

Personality and the group matrix

Sigmund Karterud, Espen Folmo and Mickey Kongerslev

Abstract

This article starts with the fact that groups are social systems and that their matrix will be affected by the nature of these systems, for example, that it needs energy to keep them going. Without this energy, groups will dissolve, i.e., lose their boundaries and disappear in the surrounding community. E.g., psychotherapy groups might lose their defining characteristics and turn into common social gatherings. Where is this energy coming from? We argue that it comes from the SEEKING system of the therapist, dependent on his/her dopamine activation, and cultivated by his/her theoretical, relational and technical knowledge. Since the task of the group is self- and personality development of the group members, it requires theoretical knowledge about the vicissitudes of the self and personality, and how these phenomena become intertwined in the ongoing group discourse, i.e., the matrix. We briefly outline the TAM theory of personality, and through a video-taped case study, we demonstrate how the therapists succeed in engaging a reluctant group member in a group discourse which become meaningful to all members and thus permeates the matrix. However, during the last part of the group, it punctuates, loses its energy and can hardly be distinguished from a café gathering. The matrix and the group processes related to it, undergo a radical change. By this case study we illuminate how the quality of the group matrix is related to e.g., the therapists theoretical understanding of borderline and attachment dynamics and the therapist's competence in initiating a mentalizing discourse that engage all members in the group.

The concept of group matrix

As a way of introduction: S. H. Foulkes coined the central concepts of group analysis, of which the most important was the *group matrix*: "the cornerstone of our working theory" (Foulkes & Anthony, 1957: 217). In Foulkes' terminology, matrix refers to the relatedness/communion and established communicational web or network that exists among people who are united for some purpose (Foulkes, 1990).

DOI: 10.4324/9781003625810-9

He distinguished between the foundation matrix and the dynamic matrix. The foundation matrix refers to the part of the communicational network that stems from our common biological makeup, our senses, our capacity for linguistic communication as well as our particular type of language and culture. The dynamic matrix refers to the on-going and fluctuating communicational network in a particular group situated in a certain context and constituted by some specific needs and/or purposes. That said, Foulkes never provided us with a clear and concise working definition of the matrix, but rather left a legacy of various suggestive and evocative descriptions throughout his oeuvre (Ahlin, 1985). Hence, newer discourses on the matrix have sought to elaborate and clarify this key concept.

Communion and communication between group members are to a large extent dependent on unconscious processes. Thanks to the work of Hopper, the role of *social unconscious*, has become a target for fruitful contemporary exploration and discourse (Hopper, 2002, 2018). Nitzgen and Hopper (2017: 202) have suggested a tripartite nature of social systems, consisting of "three overlapping and interpenetrating matrices: the foundation matrix of the wider contextual society, the dynamic matrix of a particular grouping …, and the personal matrices of the members of a particular social entity." Moreover, Schermer, (2018) has recently emphasised four modalities of the experience of the others as basic determinants of information and feedback channels within the communication matrix. These four modalities are: Mind, body, gaze and face.

The tripartite matrix of Nitzgen and Hopper (2017) is formulated as a general individual-group-society theory, while Schermer (2018) also specifies some implications for clinical group analysis. Though these theoretical contributions enrich the discourse on the matrix, we also believe that some essential components are missing. We miss reflections about the energy source of groups in a social system theory sense. But most of all, we miss reflections about the significance of personality, including emotionality. The "personal matrices" need to be specified.

In the following, we will outline the key constituents of a modern theory of personality and explicate its implications for group matrix dynamics, with special reference to therapeutic groups and the personal matrices in Nitzgen and Hopper's (2017) terms. In their efforts to build a truly social theory, prominent group analytic scholars might have neglected the individual somewhat, the personalities which make up each and every group and so profoundly contributes to its dynamic matrix (Karterud, 2011). Moreover, a thorough understanding of the group members' personality is needed, considering that personality change and development are the ultimate aims of therapeutic groups, and because we, as group therapists, are not treating groups but individuals in and through the group. Extrapolating from psychotherapy research, primarily in the modality of individual therapy, highlighting the importance of therapist effects (Wampold & Imel, 2015), we would argue that the group conductor is key in order to run an effective group that brings about personality change to its members. To illustrate our point, we analyse a clinical case. Firstly, however, we comment upon the issue of energy and social systems.

Social systems, energy and entropy

Foulkes referred to groups and matrix as "social systems" several times throughout his work (Nitzgen & Hopper, 2017), but to our knowledge he did not discuss the topic of energy. Social systems, however, are loaded with energy that fuel their purposive actions and boundary maintenance. There is no energy source in social systems as such, except for the contribution by each single member, in interaction with others. A productive group succeeds in releasing energy from its members for the benefit of common goals and purposes. But what is the nature of this energy? Spinoza called it *conatus*, Freud *libido*, and the neuroscientist Damasio *homeostatic energy* or *feelings*. We find Panksepp's conceptualization to be most congruent with the currently available scientific data (Panksepp, 1998; Panksepp & Biven, 2012). He labels it SEEKING, i.e. a primary emotional system that drives organisms to pursue their goals. Dopamine is the central neurotransmitter in the seeking system. Provide dopamine to mammals, and they will keep going with their business, boasted with energy. If dopamine is blocked, they will become lethargic. Accordingly, if groups are to succeed with their endeavours, they must arouse the seeking system of its members.

Part of the energy must be invested in maintenance of group boundaries. In nature, energy differences between interacting systems are regulated by the second law of thermodynamics, which implies a tendency towards increasing entropy, which means less organised differences between systems (Magnavita, 2005). Ultimately, the whole universe moves towards chaos. All organised differences will be levelled out. This entropy tendency must be counteracted, e.g., by investing in boundary maintenance of systems. It is debatable whether the principle of entropy is applicable to social systems (Bailey, 1990). However, it has heuristic value. If social systems do not invest energy in boundary maintenance and renewal of their identity scripts and purposes, their delineation and differences compared to competing social systems/scripts will decrease, and they will cease to exist or be left to survive as petrified anomalies.

The purpose of clinical group analysis is to promote personality change and development among its members. To succeed with this goal, group analysis must create and maintain a certain (therapeutic) group climate and discourse – a specific type of dynamic matrix. The group analyst is the key agent and energizing source in this project. S/he strives to realise something that resembles an ideal group discourse, which s/he has in his/her mind. Key factors in the process are the group analysts own personality, training, clinical experience, and theoretical understanding. S/he has invested significant energy to reach at that point where s/he feels qualified to set up a therapeutic group. The crucial point now is that s/he must use that knowledge and energy to counteract the conventional type of conversational discourse that the group members carry with them as their "default mode". Left alone, group members will tend to gravitate towards conventional talk. That is how entropy can affect the group discourse. The group needs someone who has the knowledge, skills and energy to counteract this, and make a difference. A crucial component of this knowledge base is the therapist's theory of personality, which we will turn to next. It is our impression that the "personal matrices of the members" are somewhat neglected in the theory of group analysis. For example, Nitzgen and Hopper (2017) devote far more attention to the foundation and dynamic matrix. Admittedly, those aspects are more "groupish", but when it comes to clinical group analysis, it is after all the personality of the members we work with, as they interact in and with the group/other members and therapists.

Broadly speaking, we suggest that (a) enhanced affect consciousness, (b) improved interpersonal competences, including a more secure and trustful attachment pattern, together with (c) more robust and sophisticated mentalization are the most central domains involved in positive personality change in therapeutic groups. In the therapeutic group setting, members cannot help but react emotionally towards each other; each of the members characteristic attachment orientation/interpersonal style will materialise in the here and now, as well as their mentalizing abilities in terms of making sense of self, others and the group. Thus, the group analyst needs to know the basics of the members' personality, as it provides the foundation for understanding each member in the group, and their continuous contribution to the dynamic matrix, as well the central domains that needs to change.

The temperament-attachment-mentalizing (TAM) theory of personality

To further our understanding of personality we have recently outlined a new theory that highlights three major constituents: Temperament (mainly primary emotions), attachment and self-consciousness (mentalizing) (Karterud, 2017; Karterud & Kongerslev, 2018; Karterud & Kongerslev, 2019). The constituents are dynamically interrelated in the individual and come in the following evolutionary order: Temperament comes first, and is a prerequisite for attachment, which in turn preludes mentalizing. Furthermore, we argue that the elements of temperament have undergone natural selection according to established evolutionary principles. Attachment has some features that link it to temperament, but the typical attachment orientation of the individual is mainly a product of early experiences. Mentalizing is an ability that develops within the context of attachment relationships and entails the ability to understand self and other as psychological beings with intentions as well as the internalization of cultural achievements and codes. Thus, there appears to be a movement in our species' socio-cultural history and in the ontogenesis of the individual subject, from nature (evolution) to intersubjective learning, symbolization and cultural internalization (socio-cultural processes). Individuals are shaped in different and distinctive ways by the dynamics of these intricate processes. We elaborate.

Temperament is the evolutionary oldest part of personality. Homo sapiens share with all mammals the following seven primary emotional systems: SEEKING,

FEAR, RAGE, (sexual) LUST, SEPARATION DISTRESS (sadness), CARE (love) and PLAY (joy) (Panksepp & Biven, 2012). Considering that there is motion in e-motion, these seven primary emotional systems have evolved as responses to evolutionary adaptive challenges, and they are powerful motivators for action. Apart from the primary emotions, we also consider *effortful control* (MacDonald, 2008; Posner & Rothbart, 1998), *conscientiousness* (McCrae & Costa, 2003), and *dominance/social rank behaviour* (Qu et al., 2017) as part of temperament.

Individuals are highly different with respect to consciousness of their (primary) emotions as well as these emotions' trigger levels, intensity when activated, tolerance of experiencing them, and the ability to regulate them. Personality disorders have their distinct temperamental profiles in terms of primary emotional traits (Karterud et al., 2016). For example, separation distress and rage are the most difficult emotions for individuals with borderline personality disorder, while people with a narcissistic inclination are particularly driven by social rank behaviour. These sensitivities will manifest themselves in groups. The temperaments, in themselves, fuel the group with energy. Foremost is the exploratory SEEKING system. To quote Panksepp (1998, p. 52), the SEEKING system:

> … makes animals intensely interested in exploring their world and leads them to become excited when they are about to get what they desire. It eventually allows animals to find and eagerly anticipate the things they need for survival … When fully aroused, it helps fill the mind with interest and motivates organisms to move … in search of the things they need, crave, and desire. In humans, this may be one of the main brain systems that generate and sustain curiosity, even for intellectual pursuits.

Attachment presupposes the primary emotions of FEAR and SEPARATION DISTRESS, which, when activated in children, trigger CARE behaviour among parents. These temperamental dispositions are thus prerequisites for attachment behaviour, which, when repeated a multitude of times, foster the attachment pattern of the child, and thereby the organizing templates for later interpersonal relatedness. As we know, attachment patterns have a decisive influence upon the course of life and truly count as a personality qualifier (Levy et al., 2015). Most patients in groups in the National Health Services have insecure attachment patterns and these patterns will manifest themselves in the group and influence the dynamic matrix (Karterud, 2011). For borderline patients it concerns primarily anxious-ambivalent and disorganised attachment. One important goal of group therapies is to amend the attachment patterns and improve relational competence.

Mentalization presupposes both primary emotions and attachment. While several of man's emotional proclivities can be traced back to neurobiological developments around 500 million years ago, mentalization is a cultural achievement of fairly new origin, e.g., 100–200.000 years ago. Mentalization also presupposes language and communication, and is the internalization in the individual of signs, symbols, meaning and narratives that have been sanctioned by the group to which one belongs (Tomasello, 2014). Foulkes adopted this view at an early stage (Foulkes & Anthony, 1957). However, it was only after his time that researchers established that mentalization was a dimensional affair; some excels at it, while others have poor abilities. Further it was found that mentalizing abilities was dependent on the individual's attachment experiences, including attachment traumas and faulty mirroring, and linked to psychopathology (Bateman & Fonagy, 2016; Bo et al., 2017). Accordingly, another important goal of group therapy is to increase the ability to process painful experiences and interpersonal difficulties, as well as stabilizing and improving the group participants ability to mentalise.

The TAM-theory and the matrix

The TAM theory adds more specificity to the tripartite matrix as conceived by Nitzgen and Hopper (2017). The group members' diverse temperaments coin the foundation and dynamic matrix. In groups of other mammals than Homo sapiens, members CARE about each other, they PLAY together, and they react with SEPARATION DISTRESS. They FEAR predators, display RAGE towards intruders, and have sex due to the primary emotional system of LUST. Above all, they stick together as a group because of attachment. Also, other mammals than Homo sapiens perform in this foundational matrix in individualised ways, attesting to 'personal matrices'. Some go for an alpha-male position, while others subordinate. There is a lively social unconscious activity in e.g., primate groups when power struggle goes on, or when allies groom each other.

Schermer (2018: 179) is concerned with how persons experience each other in groups: "The *Mind* thinks about other minds; the *Body* feels its way into others' emotions; the *Gaze* express power and control, and the *Face* demands recognition and care". Translated into TAM-theory, we would say: The mind mentalizes; empathy is dependent on CARE, power and control is fuelled by dominance and social rank behaviour; FEAR and SEPARATION DISTRESS (displayed by the face) appeals to CARE. Schermer writes very informatively on how Western philosophers have conceptualised issues related to mind, body, gaze and face. However, we prefer that this becomes rooted in and supplemented with more rigorous empirical research including the life sciences; this will increase the explanatory power.

Today we have good scientific theories that can explain how the dynamic matrix of a particular therapeutic group will be profoundly shaped by the personality characteristics of the members. E.g., the more severe borderline pathology, the more unstable membership. The more separation anxiety and rage, the more instances of breakdowns in mentalizing. The more narcissistic the members are, the more power-struggle and pseudo-mentalization, and the less care. The more avoidant the patients are, the more fear and less curious exploration and play. In the following, we will illustrate our proposition with case material from a therapeutic group.

Case illustration

The group was a long term, slow open outpatient group for personality disorders at the Department of Personality Psychiatry, Oslo University Hospital. The group was conducted according to modified group-analytic principles and consisted of one male and five female members with severe personality disorders, mostly of a borderline type. Both of the two group therapists were qualified group analysts. The group was video-recorded in 2006 as part of a research project and was conserved for later scrutiny and comparisons with other type of groups. The group discourse was transcribed to a text covering 21 pages. All participants, patients and therapists, gave their consent to the research project that was approved by the regional ethical committee. The authors analysed the group in 2018, when this group was included in a larger study that compared this type of group therapy with mentalization-based group therapy (MBT-G) (Karterud, 2015).

The first ten minutes in this group was filled with the therapists' (T-1 and T-2) focus on absences from the group and in particular on patient-3 (P-3) who told that she could not attend the group regularly because of insufficient money for public transport. The therapists expressed concern for her lack of money, but also tried to explore other possible motives, and her priorities in money affairs. P-3 stated repeatedly that the issue here was poverty – period: There were no feelings involved and no hidden motives! Eventually the therapists gave in, and they turned to patient-4:

T-1: *Eh – something different … we have thought … the co-therapist and I … and talked about, the last sessions, how you … yes, how you … how has it been for you being in the group, what you have done with or used the group for, and thought that … in a way you have said that you have become more and more depressed.*

To this kind invitation to speak about her mental state (depressed) in the group, P-4 confirms the label depressed,

> … yes, but what can I do about it, I don't know.

She says that she is crying most of the time, can't do anything, and points to her chest where she says there is a "cramped fist".

T-1 supports and encourage her to speak about it in the group, refers to another group member who also was depressed recently and where the group was engaged in finding out what were the circumstances, what triggered the episode and what could possibly maintain it. Patient-1 and P-2 support T-1 in trying to engage P-4. P-4 responds in a way that signals a very low level of mentalizing:

"No, I don't think … I cannot bear to talk about it", "Yes, but I don't know what I shall … No, I believe I am very vulnerable now, in all respects, I believe so".

T-1 proceeds with telling what everybody knew:

But to have … you have talked very little about to be affected … or the fact that you have got a cancer disease, and you have received chemotherapy … Nothing has been your fault. You have been struck by it. How is it to be in the group, when at the same time having suffered that much but shared so little of your experiences? …

P-4: *Yes, but … I believe the worst thing is what happened to John (boyfriend). The lack of empathy and understanding he has displayed. … Concerning … expressing feelings and despair and such things. He will not lis … he will not listen to that. It's like what you [T-1] have said earlier, he has no empathy. That's the toughest part of it. He has not even hugged me when we have gone to bed, never held me, nothing. Now when I have been ill. It has been … painful.*

T-1: *It sounds horrible and painful if you ask me. And in the group, you have not been hugged either, not in a physical sense, but we might have given you another type of care, or how have you perceived that?*

P-4: *I have received very little here … But he thinks I complain too much, see? So … I am not allowed to think other thoughts than everything is going to be fine, that I should be fine. Oh … he is horrible, it is horrible.*

T-1: *But being so dismissive, P-4, when it comes to the group, when people here actually have approached you …*

P-4: *Yes, but I don't want to burst, see? Because it is such a huge abscess to penetrate, and if I started to talk about such things, it would pour out …*

T-1: *However, at the same time, you are longing for some more … eh … empathy concerning … your situation? And it is … what you fear with that bursting … what is it more precisely?*

P-4: *I hate sitting here crying. It's so much … it's so much that … While I'm sitting here, it might also concern patient Mary in the group …"*

We see here, from the transcript, that P-4 starts out with a very low reflective functioning (RF), in the range of zero: *"… I cannot bear to talk about it"*. The resistance continues through the discourse, e.g., she fears a breakdown. However, therapist T-1 pressures her gently, being emphatic but also challenging: *"… what is it more precisely?"*. P-4 then enters a long narrative of increasing complexity and nuances, lasting for nearly an hour, starting with fellow patient Mary in the group (absent this session). P-4 has got it that Mary can't stand strong feelings in the group, and another complication is that she lives in P-4's neighbourhood. If Mary gets to know details of her private life, and all the stuff about John, P-4 would feel invaded, losing the neighbourhood as a space of her own. From now on the other group members get more and more involved in the story of P-4. They ask her relevant questions, support her, displays empathy, and challenge her. Fellow patients supply the story with small excursions into own life experiences, but thereafter return to P-4. The theme of Mary dissipates soon, and the main theme becomes P-4's pain and needs in her difficult life situation and the poor relationship to John. Increasingly, the relationship to the group enters the main stage. The therapists act as the main players in the background. As the story unfolds in the group, it is by no means linear. It is messy, sometimes confusing, but the therapists act as a sort of anchor or compass, helping to bring the discourse back to the main track, which concerns P-4's attachment pattern that prevents her from finding mental nourishment where it actually resides.

T-1: *When I think about your relation to us, P-4, here in the group, there's people here which you can make use of, but you tend to reject that, the contacts here. I wonder why. I try to understand why you do that. Because you are now telling how much you need closeness, care and concern, but you reject.*

P-4 responds by exploring more of her intersubjective transactions with others, her fear that other people (e.g., in the group), might despise her, find her egocentric, but how can she know what other people feel and think (?), and then she reflects about the responsibility of taking the centre stage. If she did, things would become more real in a way. Others, and she herself, might start to expect that she takes things more seriously, that she starts a process of change, and what if she does not succeed? However, she appreciates that the group, this time, has pushed her:

> I really appreciate what you are doing now. I realize that I have been sending signals about it, that I want it, but at the same time I don't want it.

During this one-hour group therapy sequence, we can observe a marked increase in the reflective functioning of P-4, from a rather non-mentalizing functioning ("I cannot bear to talk about it"), to a definitely more complex, sophisticated and psychologically meaningful reflection about own emotions, thoughts, interpersonal transactions, self-understanding and understanding of others. At the same time, it can be demonstrated how this increase in mentalizing capacity is embedded in a group discourse that is characterised by engagement from all group members and emotional resonance with diverse and multiple perspectives, however, oscillating around an axis of reflection about her attachment difficulties by exploring her relationship to the group here and now. It is also clear how the "group machine", so to speak, got started, with energy input from the therapists – they successfully stimulated the members SEEKING system.

The preceding paragraph describes the group matrix. Everybody is involved in the communicational web. After the "kick-start" from the therapists, it might seem like the group was almost self-going. However, scrutiny of the video and the transcript revealed that the therapists provided several interventions along the course that kept the group "on track". And this "on track" seems to be linked to the energy source that fuels a highly meaningful, vital and engaged discourse. Being "on track" implies that the theme resonates with important attachment experiences and emotions among most group members. As these painful attachment experiences are associated with a diversity of defensive strategies, shared by most of the group members, it could easily lead the group astray in the absence the therapists' efforts. The energy released into the group matrix, the communicational flow, the content of what is communicated, the ability to reflect upon it, and the emotional awareness and attunement, in short, the quality of the group matrix, was dependent on the therapists' capacities and theoretical understanding of insecure and disorganised attachment, the significance of attachment traumas for borderline personality disorder, the intolerance of separation distress and the disastrous consequences of the rage coupled with it, combined with technical skills in how to handle the transference manifestation of it in groups that contain many borderline patients.

The topic of the matrix becomes all the more important when we follow this group through the last 30 minutes of the session. Something peculiar happens. It is the same group, the same people who previously engaged in a highly charged and meaningful group interaction. However, after one hour, the group matrix undergoes a profound change.

The theme changes to general concerns, like how much one should work, is it good for one's mental health, what if it drains all one's energy, and how much should one socialise with other people? Most group members engage in this discussion, including T-2 who previously was quite silent. However, the quality of the communication in the group matrix is now very different. It is as if nothing serious is at stake any longer. Not that the conversation is meaningless, but it lacks a nerve, it lacks energy. It's a type of conversation that could have taken place among ordinary Norwegian people meeting for a chat in a shopping mall. They share opinions about this and that. The therapists pose some questions about how it is to socialise with other group members after the session, but they are not followed up in any sense, they are not part of a therapeutic strategy of the same sort as we observed in the first sequence. It is as if the therapists had been drained of all energy, as if their SEEKING system had been turned off, which sets the stage for entropy to take over. Indeed, optimal arousal (not too low nor to high) is a prerequisite for optimal mentalizing, which in turn is a prerequisite for the members to become engaged in the therapeutic project (Bateman & Fonagy, 2016). From this perspective, the session also demonstrates how the group therapists initially manage to find an optimal arousal/anxiety level in the group that allows for the group members to become engaged and explore each other's minds and relations, whereas towards the end, the arousal level dropped and mentalizing got turned down.

Discussion

One may argue that the therapeutic style of this group was too "authority-centred" and too less "sibling/group-centred" to be of relevance for group analytic theory. However, this impression may be exaggerated since the transcript citations in the paragraph above mainly contain interactions between the dominant group therapist and patient-4. However, this selection is done for didactic purposes (and space limitations). As we write in the text, everybody was "involved in the communicational web. After the "kick-start" from the therapists, it might seem like the group was almost self-going". The two group therapists were qualified group analysts, and their professional self-understanding was that they conducted "modified group analytic psychotherapy" for a selected group of severely disordered patients. Moreover, group matrices are not reserved for group analytic groups. Important insights may come from other than "classical" analytic groups.

One reviewer of this paper commented that the concept of personality is not identical to "personal matrix". We very much agree. Personality is defined by the relatively stable emotional, relational and cognitive characteristics of the individual. Personality has more to do with process and structure, than phenomenal content. By contrast, personal matrix will include the unique experiential world of the individual. Thus, we claim that the structures and processes of personality often exert deeper influence on the group matrix than personal matrix alone. In our case report, the personal matrix of P-4 involved bitter resentment and withdrawal with particular references to her boyfriend John. However, we would say that these phenomena were contingent upon a deeper and unconscious insecure attachment pattern. The last statement of course implies a theoretical understanding of the individual. We contend that group analysts should be sensitive to the personal matrix as it evolves in the here and now, but at the same time search for a theoretical understanding according to modern personality theory.

One may also argue that what we define as "personality change and development", is not necessarily the aim of group analysis. It may be better conceptualised as "better communication, more satisfaction with life and to fully fulfil our potentials as individuals" (reviewer comment). Here, we think, we are in the midst of an important debate for group analysis. Is group analysis primarily a theory and practice for middle class people (e.g., health professionals) that strive to enhance their quality of life, or is it a treatment for patients in the NHS? It might be both, but we would argue that if it loses terrain as an efficient clinical modality for treatment seeking people, it will be marginalised. Admittedly, most (real) patients do not seek psychotherapy for openly admitted concern about their "personality". But if one listens to most complaints, they are related to poor emotional consciousness, dysfunctional interpersonal patterns and mentalizing dysfunction. That is, according to our view, personality problems par excellence.

A final issue concerns our interpretation of the last 30 minutes, which we have characterised as "ordinary conversation". We do not say that the group has "regressed" or something in that direction. What we observed in this group case was first a sequence where the therapists eventually succeeded in activating most members in a productive exchange that normal social conventions would not stimulate. However, this sequence was then followed by a group discourse that was different, and hardly distinguishable from everyday talk. There was a distinct change in the matrix, and this should be explained. Different explanations will have different explanatory power. We have suggested an explanation that combines modern personality theory with group dynamics and social systems theory.

As we argued in the introduction, social systems need energy and a certain structure in order to resist the principle of entropy. Hence, psychotherapy groups must be infused with energy, communicative rules, and professional theory and ideals in order for it to avoid an everyday discourse. The sources of such structures, or energy, are of course diverse, but in order to navigate the matrix in a way that turns its discourse into a transformative vehicle, it seems that therapists need a compass of alliance and strategy in combination with a willingness to confront the members' comfort zone in a skilful and tailored manner.

Somewhat contrary to this view, one may argue that groups simply need a pause, now and then, from highly emotionally charged sequences. That is a valid point of view. It may be that the group needs to "digest" what it has experienced, in order to move forward again. We do not exclude such an interpretation. However, that view does not alter the phenomena of a striking change in the group matrix. Well into the calm conversational phase of the group, the group therapist in this case might have commented: "The atmosphere in the group seems calmer now, while it was highly emotionally charged when you were in the centre, P-4. Are these phenomena related? Was it necessary with a pause in some way?" However, if such an interpretation is valid, it actually confirms the views we have expressed on group matrix, energy and entropy.

Concluding remarks

We find the contribution of Nitzgen and Hopper (2017) about the "tripartite" nature of the matrix as most important. The three constituents of the matrix are of course interrelated. In this article we have suggested that the significance of the personality constituent has been underestimated in group analytic theory. We have outlined a modern theory of personality which integrates temperament, attachment and self-consciousness, and analysed a group case where one of the group members displayed gross problems with primary emotions (particularly separation distress), attachment behaviour and mentalizing. We hopefully succeeded in demonstrating how this particular "personal matrix" interacted with and influenced the group as a whole (dynamic matrix). The elements of interpersonal sensitivity and separation anxiety, the anxious-ambivalent attachment and the low mentalizing ability set the tone for the group discourse. Thanks to competent group therapists, the initial resistance was overcome, and the group did an impressive piece of psychotherapeutic work. It was marked in the end of the sequence when the main protagonist expressed gratitude to the group. The case highlights the importance of personality theory for understanding the interrelatedness of personal matrices and the dynamic matrix. We would even maintain that the personality theory is valid for explaining and understanding important elements of the foundation matrix, its evolutionary heritage or natural history and bio-psycho-social underpinnings, in human and other mammal groups, as we are all destined by the dynamic interplay of primary emotions and attachment behaviour. Destined, however, as we might be by these forces which makes our nature, there is also a bit of freedom bestowed upon us through our mentalizing capacities, which allows us to reflect upon ourselves, others and society and to some extent intentionally work on changing our actions and reactions. But that is another story about other aspects of personal matrices and the group matrix.

References

Ahlin, G. (1985). On thinking about the group matrix. *Group Analysis,* 18(2): 111–119.

Bailey, K. D. (1990). *Social Entropy Theory.* New York: SUNY Press.

Bateman, A. & Fonagy, P. (2016). *Mentalization-Based Treatment for Personality Disorders: A Practical Guide.* Oxford: Oxford University Press.

Bo, S., Sharp, C., Fonagy, P. et al. (2017). Hypermentalizing, attachment, and epistemic trust in adolescent BPD: Clinical illustrations. *Personality Disorders* 8(2): 172–182.

Foulkes, S. H. (1990). The group as matrix of the individual's mental life. In E. Foulkes (Ed.), *S. H. Foulkes Selected Papers: Psychoanalysis and Group Analysis.* London: Karnac Books.

Foulkes, S. H. & Anthony, E. J. (1957). *Group Psychotherapy: The Psychoanalytic Approach.* London: Penguin Books.

Hopper, E. (2002). *The Social Unconscious: Selected Papers.* London: Jessica Kingsley Publishers.

Hopper, E. (2018). The development of the concept of the Tripartite Matrix: A response to 'Four modalities of the experience of others in groups' by Victor Schermer. *Group Analysis,* 51(2): 197–206.

Karterud, S. (2011). Constructing and mentalizing the matrix. *Group Analysis,* 44(4): 357–373.

Karterud, S. (2015). *Mentalization-Based Group Therapy (MBT-G): A Theoretical, Clinical, and Research Manual.* Oxford: Oxford University Press.

Karterud, S. (2017). *Personlighet.* Oslo: Gyldendal.

Karterud, S. & Kongerslev, M. T. (2019). A temperament-attachment-mentalization-based (TAM) theory of personality and its disorders. *Frontiers of Psychology,* 10. https://doi.org/10.3389/fpsyg.2019.00518

Karterud, S. & Kongerslev, M. T. (2019). Case formulations in mentalization-based treatment (MBT) for patients with borderline personality disorder. In U. Kramer (Ed.), *Case Formulation for Personality Disorders: Tailoring Psychotherapy to the Individual Client.* Oxford: Academic Press.

Karterud, S., Pedersen, G., Johansen, M. et al. (2016). Primary emotional traits in patients with personality disorders. *Personality and Mental Health,* 10(4): 261–273.

Levy, K. N., Johnson, B. N., Clouthier, T. L. et al. (2015). An attachment theoretical framework for personality disorders. *Canadian Psychology,* 56(2): 197–207.

MacDonald, K. B. (2008). Effortful control, explicit processing, and the regulation of human evolved predispositions. *Psychological Review,* 115(4): 1012–1031.

Magnavita, J. J. (2005). Systems theory foundations of personality, psychopathology, and psychotherapy. In S. Strack (Ed.), *Handbook of Personology and Psychopathology.* Hoboken: Wiley.

McCrae, R. R. & Costa, P. T. (2003). *Personality in Adulthood: A Five Factor Theory Perspective.* New York: Guilford Press.

Nitzgen, D. & Hopper, E. (2017). The concepts of the social unconscious and of the matrix in the work of S. H. Foulkes. In E. Hopper & H, Weinberg (Eds.), *The Social Unconsciousness in Persons, Groups, and Societies: The Foundation Matrix Extended and Re-Configured.* London: Karnac Books.

Panksepp, J. (1998). *Affective Neuroscience: The Foundations of Human and Animal Emotions.* Oxford: Oxford University Press.

Panksepp, J. & Biven, L. (2012). *The Archaeology of Mind: Neuroevolutionary Origins of Human Emotions.* New York: W. W. Norton & Company.

Posner, M. I. & Rothbart, M. K. (1998). Attention, self-regulation and consciousness. *Philosophical Transactions of the Royal Society of London, Series B, Biological Sciences,* 353: 1915–1927.

Qu, C., Ligneul, R., Van der Henst, J. B. et al. (2017). An integrative interdisciplinary perspective on social dominance hierarchies. *Trends in Cognitive Sciences,* 21(11): 893–908.

Schermer, V. L. (2018). Four modalities of the experience of others in groups. *Group Analysis,* 51(2): 175–196.

Tomasello, M. (2014). *A Natural History of Human Thinking.* Cambridge: Harvard University Press.

Wampold, B. E. & Imel, Z. E. (2015). *The Great Psychotherapy Debate: The Evidence for What Makes Psychotherapy Work.* London: Routledge.

Chapter 10

On the relationship between group analysis and mentalization-based group therapy

Sigmund Karterud, Gordon Gunnarsen, Mickey Kongerslev, Lenka Staun, and Ulrich Schultz-Venrath

Abstract

In this article we describe and reflect upon the roots of mentalization-based group therapy (MBT-G) and its relationship to group analysis. The original setting for MBT was psychotherapeutic day hospitals that were strongly influenced by group analytic thinking. The challenges from an increasing number of borderline patients initiated theoretical and therapeutic innovations that separated MBT-G from traditional group analysis who responded differently, e.g., by strengthening its ties to object-relational theories that emphasised innate destructive drives. Since then, the dialogue between the two approaches have been meagre in the UK, but more constructive in e.g., Norway and Germany. We argue that MBT- G needs group analytic competence with respect to basic group dynamics, and that group analysis needs revitalization by the theory of mentalizing. We call for dialogues between the two approaches. The authors belong to both camps and speak with reference to experiences in Norway, United Kingdom, Denmark and Germany.

Breeding grounds of MBT-G

The breeding grounds of mentalization-based group therapy (MBT-G) were psychotherapeutic day hospitals, strongly influenced by therapeutic community ideology and group analysis (Bateman & Fonagy, 1999; Karterud et al., 1992). The most important sites were St. Ann's Hospital in London where the day treatment programme was directed by Anthony Bateman, and Oslo University Hospital (OUS) where the day treatment programme was directed by Sigmund Karterud. These treatment programmes were composed of a wide range of group therapies and the theoretical matrix that sustained them was influenced by authors such as S. H. Foulkes, Tom Main, Maxwell Jones, Wilfred Bion, Henry Ezriel, Pat de Maré and others. In the early 2000s, these programmes were converted to

DOI: 10.4324/9781003625810-10

intensive outpatient treatment programmes composed of 1) an introductory psychoeducational group, 2) weekly individual psychotherapy and 3) weekly group psychotherapy. By that reduction, the group component lost its embeddedness in theories and practice of communal living and learning (Foulkes, 1948). It is noteworthy that the first practical MBT guidelines, published in 2006, lacked any reference to group analytic theory (Bateman & Fonagy, 2006). However, most of the MBT group therapists of that generation brought with them at least some kind of group analytic training. E.g., when the programme at Oslo University Hospital converted from day hospital to intensive outpatient treatment in 2008, most group therapists were qualified group analysts. The new theories of MBT (Bateman & Fonagy, 2006) were thus integrated with a preexisting corpus of group analytic theory and practice.

The connection between MBT-G and group analysis become diluted in the UK

In the years to come, on the international scene, the original connection between group analysis (GA) and MBT was diluted. The group component of MBT was treated as the stepchild of the approach. In the next MBT treatment guidelines (Bateman & Fonagy, 2016) the group component was given somewhat more consideration (38 pages). However, the chapter was completely uncontextualised. Except for Bion (1961), there was no reference whatsoever to any group psychotherapy literature. Since this second treatment guidelines, Bateman & Fonagy have published two articles on MBT group therapy yet still without relating the MBT group approach to the world of group analysis and psychodynamic group psychotherapy (Bateman, Kongerslev, & Hansen, 2019; Fonagy, Campbell, & Bateman, 2017). This relative lack of integrating the theoretical heritage has been paralleled by a lack of extensive training in MBT group therapy. On the advanced course of MBT at the Anna Freud Centre, minimal time (around one hour) is allocated to the MBT group component. There is no further training in MBT group therapy in the UK. It goes without saying that when MBT group therapists formerly trained in group analysis are dying out, MBT will be facing a rather large problem. Therapists with no formal group psychotherapy training, and neither with any substantial formal MBT group training, are therefore expected to (learn to) handle the most complicated group dynamics through personal experience and supervision alone. Thus, we argue there is a need for more dedicated and lengthy training in MBT-G.

A different course in Norway and Germany

The course in Norway and Germany have been different. Textbooks have been written (Karterud, 2012; Karterud, 2015a; Schultz-Venrath & Felsberger, 2016), MBT-G research have been conducted as well as specialised training. The most comprehensive training in MBT-G is probably found in Norway. The Norwegian Institute for Mentalization has offered courses (consisting of 8 one-day seminars throughout a year) in MBT-G since 2008. Around 200 therapists have been trained so far. Some of the participants have had previous group analytic training, others have not. The participants are obliged to run a MBT group where most of the patients have a severe personality disorder and discuss video-recordings of this group throughout the year. In addition to theoretical discussions, there is a strong emphasis on roleplay in MBT-groups where the participants rotate in the role of therapists. Through this setup, the participants are obliged to identify with low emotional consciousness, insecure attachment patterns and mentalizing deficits. Thereby the groups are filled with non-mentalised emotions and relational obscurities and the (rotating) group therapists are faced with all kinds of primitive defences and acting out. The MBT-G trainer will observe the group from outside the circle for around 45–60 minutes and thereafter direct the lively discussions that follow on all kind of issues, from dynamics of the individuals to group dynamics, appropriate and not so appropriate interventions, missed opportunities, authority issues, arousal levels, handling of non-mentalizing modes and dimensions of mentalizing, interventions that went well, etc. Sometimes the MBT-G trainer will join the roleplay for modelling purposes. The elements of video-recordings and extensive roleplaying add some new dimensions to traditional group psychotherapy training and favour detailed technical and theoretical discussions. In comparison, group analytic training has traditionally relied more on written notes and narratives from the trainees.

In Norway, MBT group training has also been provided by the Institute of Group Analysis in Oslo. The prerequisites here are that participants have fulfilled the first introductory year of group psychotherapy and that they are enrolled in one of the subsequent courses. Accordingly, these participants partake in a dual track, both training in group-analytic psychotherapy (GA) and MBT-G. The GA training in Norway is a block training that consists of five three-day "blocks" each year. There is added one extra day for the MBT-G trainees, and their course consists of ten one day seminars over two years.

In Germany, so far MBT-G training have taken place in weekend courses that are not yet fully standardised. A popular attraction has been group therapy slams on stage, where once a year different group therapies are compared with role plays by psychotherapists during the Lindau Psychotherapy Weeks. However, currently interesting changes are taking place. In Germany, two institutes have been founded in 2021 and 2022, MBT-D-A-CH (D for Germany, A for Austria and CH for Switzerland) in Heidelberg and IGAM (Institute for Group Analysis and Mentalizing in Groups) in Cologne/Muenster. Both are in the process of developing a curriculum for MBT-G and mentalizing in groups. Likewise, a MBT-G focus is currently being established at the International Psychoanalytic University (IPU) Berlin. As a GA and MBT-G-therapist, Lenka Staun has set up an IPU group therapy lab that embeds extensive process and outcome research over the course of MBT-G and GA treatment. The aim of this initiative is to firmly anchor both, MBT-G and GA, with their theoretical and clinical foundations into a university institution. Moreover, the application of MBT-G is extended to the specific treatment of adults with ADHD.

Group analysis and severe personality disorders

The emergence of MBT around the millennium shift, was related to a partial stagnation of group analytic theory and practice. It is important to bear in mind the different roots of group analysis: It began in departments of psychiatry in the USA (e.g., by Trigant Burrow, Paul Schilder, Louis Wender, Alexander Wolf & Emanuel K. Schwartz) in the 20s and 30s of the last century (Schultz-Venrath, 2022), continued without reference to the American pioneers in the Northfield military hospital for soldiers with war neuroses (e.g., by Tom Main, John Rickman, Wilfred R. Bion and Sigmund H. Foulkes) (Harrison, 2000) and developed in the therapeutic community movement (Jones, 1963). As a result of the major treatment problems and lack of research data on structurally disturbed patients, the so-called Göttingen model developed in Germany in the 1970s and interpersonal group psychotherapy in Canada (Heigl-Evers & Heigl, 1973; Marziali & Munroe-Blum, 1994). The Göttingen model distinguishes between three different approaches to working with groups. Two of them are "classical" in that they are based on interaction and confrontation, with links to Bion, Foulkes, and more recently Fonagy. The third approach, (the "psychoanalytic-interactional method" (PIM) was specifically designed to treat patients with personality disorders in groups with the aim of accepting, validating and interpreting mistrust. This approach relies on confrontation and has developed a concept of interpretation as "interpersonal feedback" intended for the management of affect dysregulation and shame in groups with patients with severe personality disorders (Staats Bolm, & Dally, 2014; Staats, 2010). In a slightly different form, this also applies to the interpersonal approach in groups (IPT).

Early in his career, S. H. Foulkes practiced combined group and individual therapy for patients with more severe personality pathology. During the 1960-ies, the Group Analytic Practice in London became the headquarter of group analysis, with its emphasis on twice-a-week groups instead of combined psychotherapy. Group analysis became dominated by the needs, ethos and discourse of private practice, at the expense of the needs of public health services and the research community. During the 1980-ies and 1990-ies, personality disorders surfaced as professional challenges and major sources of personal and communal suffering, crystallizing around borderline personality disorder (BPD). These patients were hardly suitable for private practice but were found in groups in the public/national health mental health systems (NHS). How could group analysis cope with this challenge? The debate centred around "the difficult patient in group psychotherapy" (Roth, Stone, & Kibel, 1990) with contributions from the group analytic camp by e.g., Malcolm Pines (1990). The clinical challenge was mainly how to understand and cope with singular borderline individuals in groups. It is tempting to understand the writings of e.g., Morris Nitsun (1996 [2014]) under the same angle. Borderline patients bring with them more hatred, envy and violence, and Nitsun wrote about the naïve Foulkes that underestimated destructive forces in man. Although Foulkes had been opposed to the Kleinians and post-Kleinians (e.g., W. R. Bion) the death instinct was now afforded a more prominent position as an important "critical principle" of group analysis (Nitsun, 1996 [2014]: 146f.). However, there is an open question if group therapies in the NHS were helped or got more helpful by that reorientation.

Other aspects which were not given enough attention was the impact of loss of control of the group boundaries within the NHS. This resulted in the clinical problems of handling not only one or two borderline patients in groups, but how to conduct groups when most of the group members functioned at a borderline level. According to Foulkes' "basic law of group dynamics" (Foulkes, 1948: 29-30), collectively members of a therapeutic group should "constitute the very norm from which, individually, they deviate". This "law" is hardly valid when considering many groups in publicly funded mental health services, where those seeking help often present with significant levels of disturbance and low levels of personality functioning and collectively are at high risk of producing dysfunctional and destructive group "norms". Highly disturbed groups are likely to see harmful levels of acting out and some individual members dropping out, risking the very existence of the group, and also sometimes rendering treatment iatrogenic.

A modern understanding of "ego-training in action"

In our opinion, the return to outdated Kleinian/Bionian ideas during the 1990s was a wrong path. Elsewhere, at the same time, there was a lot of thinking, experimentation, research and discussions that were better empirically founded and that favoured new ways of thinking about personality and personality disorders. A broad range of approaches appeared, such as transference-focused psychotherapy (TFP), dialectical behavioural therapy (DBT), schema therapy (ST), and mentalization-based therapy (MBT). Several of these approaches contained a group component. However, only MBT contained a psychodynamic group. The other group approaches were basically psychoeducational or kept the focus on the individual in the group (e.g., ST).

From a group analytic point of view, the most refreshing part of MBT was that the theory (and practice) brought fresh air to Foulkes' old slogan of group analysis as "ego-training in action". What exactly does this slogan mean in the age after breakdown of ego-psychology which was the paradigm that Foulkes operated within? Dennis Brown (1994; Brown, 2006) tried to modernise it by the slogan of "self development through subjective interaction" which captured new ideas of the significance of intersubjectivity. The most important turn here was from the ego to the self, and the reliance of the self upon interaction with others, although Brown and others still lacked a coherent theory of the self. Then Peter Fonagy and coworkers (2002) came with their groundbreaking volume "Affect regulation, mentalization and the development of the self". By that, "ego-training in action" could be reformulated in a modern professional language. Foulkes had introduced the metaphor of "the group as a hall of mirrors". A modern MBT version would rather be "the group as a hall of minds and bodies". Heinz Kohut (1971) had also used the rather mechanistic concept of mirroring in his theory of self psychology. Being minded by others conveys quite other connotations than reflections in a mirror. Being minded brings hermeneutics to the foreground: Somebody conveys interpretations on what is going on in my/your mind! As children we need it desperately while we are trying to make sense of what is going on in our own mind, as well as in others and in the meeting between minds, and not at least collectively – within a group. When this trouble with making sense of, was coupled with a theory of prementalistic ways of thinking, i.e., teleological, pretend and psychic equivalence mode (Fonagy et al., 2002), it augmented the explanatory power to a significant degree. In this historical epoch, in the beginning of the 21st century, it was like the resources imbedded in object-relation theory had been exhausted. The theory had not much more to offer. But then came this theory of affect regulation, mentalization and self-development and injected a new vitality in the field by its explanatory power of borderline dynamics (Bateman & Fonagy, 2004) which could be cashed out, so to speak, in a novel kind of therapeutic discourse that even proved to be effective with an eight-year-follow-up (Bateman & Fonagy, 1999; Bateman & Fonagy, 2008) with respect to symptomatic and personality change among patients who often were stigmatised as hopelessly lost in self-destructiveness.

The MBT group discourse and its limitations

As for the group component, the MBT kind of discourse demanded a group therapist style that, above all, was more directive than the traditional group analytic. The technique of MBT-G has been outlined in several publications (Karterud, 2015a; Bateman et al., 2019; Schultz-Venrath & Felsberger, 2016; Folmo et al., 2017). Compared to GA, the purpose of the group and the role of the participants as well as the therapists are more clearly explained.

Loss of alliance and dropping out are frequent threats in groups of patients with severe personality pathology (Hummelen, Wilberg, & Karterud, 2007), and particularly in early phases of the therapeutic course of the individual. In MBT, measures are taken to support and strengthen alliance and group climate, including a concurrent introductory psychoeducational group for 8–12 sessions (MBT-I) (Bateman & Fonagy, 2016), a case formulation (Karterud, 2018), and crisis plans for individuals at risk of severe self-harm. MBT is most often delivered as a conjoint treatment with individual sessions supporting the group treatment, although stand-alone MBT-G treatments also are beginning to be tried out.

MBT-G therapists impose a certain structure to the group process (Karterud, 2015b). Firstly, MBT-G therapists engage the group in an opening phase to define a certain (albeit loose) agenda for the group session. Ideally, the topic for a group session will be out-of-group interpersonal encounters which are loaded with difficult emotions, attachment insecurity and mentalizing difficulties. The therapists assist in clarifying such events and encourage all group members to take part in explorations as to meaning and significance through so-called not-knowing stance. The same attitude is taken towards interpersonal encounters in the group and the here-and-now relevance of the participants' emotion regulation, attachment styles and mentalizing problems (as well as achievements). Overall, MBT-G therapists try to be pedagogic, avoid obscurities and "deep" interpretations; and express themselves in direct and simple ways. MBT-G therapists try to avoid misunderstandings and are helpful in clarifying them when they do occur.

MBT-G aims at "psychotherapy through the group process" (Whitaker & Lieberman, 1964) but therapists set certain limits to group associations, especially if they appear as non-mentalizing pretend mode and move into a pseudomentalizing group discursive style – an abstract and clichéd way of speaking, with seemingly psychological constructs, but devoid of more profound emotional resonance (Esposito et al., 2022). The MBT-G therapist is also concerned with creating an appropriate group culture with commonly shared norms and values, albeit not so profound as is the GA ideal. The MBT-G therapist influences the group matrix in a more explicit and authoritative way (Karterud, 2011; Inderhaug & Karterud, 2015). Above all, the MBT-G group therapist has certain strategies for controlling the group when destructive forces threaten to destroy the group or some of its members. To say it simply, the MGT-G therapist will act more as a benign but firm parental figure.

The pitfalls of the MBT-G approach might be a risk for individual therapy in groups, or a directive therapeutic style that makes the group members passive and foster submission and dependency. Another risk is that the therapists adopt a rigid version of the therapeutic guidelines and do not modify their approach according to the potentials that are embedded in a particular group at a particular time. Ideally though, MBT-G is a flexible approach. When the group culture is more mature, the MBT-G therapists may rely more on GA principles by trusting the group and letting the participants battle more on their own with sorting out relational problems in the here and now. However, such a flexible approach requires group therapists that are trained also in group-analytic theory and practice. How can we foster such an enhanced competence?

Dialogues between group analysis and MBT-G

We have traced the roots of MBT-G in group-oriented day hospitals, strongly influenced by group analytic thinking. The schism between the approaches seems to appear when persons with personality disorders, and in particular borderline personality disorder, become better identified during the 1990s and tend to dominate groups in the NHS. MBT-G develops in a direction of its own, while the response from GA is to broaden the theory with a stronger emphasis on man's supposedly innate destructiveness (Nitsun, 1996 [2014]; Schlapobersky, 2016) unrelated to borderline and antisocial personality disorders. In the short run, it seems that MBT has succeeded better with respect to borderline patients (Kvarstein et al., 2015; Hecke et al., 2016; Morken et al., 2019). However, this success is so far hardly due to any better theory of groups and group dynamics. It is mainly because of a better theory of individual personality pathology in the borderline range. When it comes to groups, there is still much to do. New progress in this field, demands in our view developments both within GA and MBT-G, and above all a better dialogue between the two.

Let's start with group analysis. As noted, we argue that GA has a weak spot when it comes to theories of personality and personality disorders. Personality is included in a vague way in the concept of matrix, which consists of a foundation matrix, a dynamic matrix and a personal matrix. However, the personal matrix is seldom discussed (Karterud, Folmo, & Kongerslev, 2019). We suggest that the very concept of matrix should be reconsidered. Could it be that it inhibits further development of GA since it limits and imprisons the individual as "a nodal point in the group matrix"? In a slogan-like way we might rather suggest: Set the individual and his/her personality free! Furthermore, is the traditional concept of the matrix too close to Foulkes's (and followers) highly speculative ideas about a "group mind"? What we miss in group analysis is a theory of "we" and "we-ness". That's what constitute a group, that *we* deliberately join forces in order to accomplish something. However, when we do that, we realise that cooperation is not an easy task. The we-ness of a therapeutic group is fundamentally coined by the personality components of the participants: What kind of emotions can we experience and reflect upon, how intimate can we be, how sophisticatedly can we reflect upon matters of concern for the individual members and the group as a whole? How can we develop our capacities for these phenomena? All group members are implicitly effected by these challenges, and they are hugely different with respect to them. There is obviously an unconscious communication going on between them. This is going on in the group self (Karterud, 1998), and may be analogue to the unconscious communication going on in the unconscious realms of the individual self, between conflicting emotions and reasoning. It is not obvious that the concept of matrix, which is rather mechanical, is the best for capturing unconscious group communication. The main problem with it is that it is impersonal, while "we" refers to "us". On the other hand, there is obviously something impersonal going on, forces that are excommunicated. Referring to Stanghellini (2017), we may label it "alterity". Psychotherapy is about participating in dialogues that tries to approach alterity, i.e., disavowed and/or hated parts of self and others. The group dialogue/polylogue or we-mode about this is what Foulkes denoted "ego-training in action". Today we may describe it as mentalizing through group interaction and reflection. Maybe we need some new concepts here, maybe not. Anthony Bateman has recently suggested a concept of "we-mode", and Wu and coworkers (2020) has proposed a somewhat speculative theory about neurobiological networks of so-called "I-mode", "Me-mode" and "We-mode". The main point is that we suggest that traditional group-analytic theories about the group has been unbalanced by overestimating the group-as-object (Nitsun, 1996) and underestimating the group-as-subject (self).

MBT-G, on the other hand, needs a more profound theory of groups and group dynamics and should lean on the more than 70 years of group analytic reflections of these basic issues. The standard MBT conception of what mentalizing consists of relies primarily on a two-person psychology of a mind that is minded by another mind. This perspective is too narrow for a proper understanding of the dialectics of the individual and the group, and society more broadly. Group analysis has the advantage of a long history of reflecting upon these questions. Unconscious realms of the group should be taken seriously and concepts like resonance (Foulkes, 1977) are paramount to an understanding of collective unconscious communication.

The basic human need for intra- and interpersonal dialogues are fully acknowledged by both parties, GA as well as MBT. We need to establish dialogues with otherness, the alien parts, in ourselves and in others. And since our practices and theories are incomplete, we need dialogues to develop our weak spots and moderate unwarranted claims. In this article we have tried to articulate some strengths and weak spots in the theory and practice of both GA and MBT-G. How can we facilitate such dialogues? Firstly, we will highlight the practice of IGA, Oslo, and IGAM (Institute of Group Analysis and Mentalizing in Groups), Köln and Münster, where courses in MBT-G and GA are arranged simultaneously. But even there, the dialogue in the teaching staff and among training candidates could be more profound. In the stricter MBT-G training, there should always be an openness for alternative views, such as "the group analytic viewpoint on this is …". On the other hand, mentalizing perspectives should be given more space in group-analytic training. Both with regard to theory and therapeutic techniques. In conferences one should try to define common themes to be discussed, e.g., "we and the matrix", "how to deal with the body mode, teleological mode, psychic equivalence and pretend mode in groups?", "conscious and unconscious cooperation", "the impact of personality on group dynamics". Seminars with strong emphasis on roleplaying might be helpful and more theoretical discussions can be arranged online for an international audience. There are abundant meeting points in a globalised world. Individuals should feel free to take initiatives here, and they should be supported by their respective institutes.

References

Bateman, A. & Fonagy, P. (2016). *Mentalization-Based Treatment for Personality Disorders – A Practical Guide.* Oxford: Oxford University Press.

Bateman, A., Kongerslev, M. & Hansen, S. B. (2019). Group therapy for adults and adolescents. In A. Bateman & P. Fonagy (Eds.), *Handbook of Mentalizing in Mental Health Practice* (pp. 117–133). Washington, DC, London, England: American Psychiatric Association Publishing.

Bateman, A. W. & Fonagy, P. (1999). Effectiveness of partial hospitalization in the treatment of borderline personality disorder: A randomized controlled trial. *American Journal of Psychiatry*, 156(10): 1563–1569.

Bateman, A. W. & Fonagy, P. (2004). *Psychotherapy for Borderline Personality Disorder. Mentalization based Treatment*. Oxford, New York: Oxford University Press.
Bateman, A. W. & Fonagy, P. (2006). *Mentalization-Based Treatment for Borderline Personality Disorder. A Practical Guide*. Oxford: Oxford University Press.
Bateman, A. W. & Fonagy, P. (2008). 8-year follow-up of patients treated for borderline personality disorder: Mentalization-based treatment versus treatment as usual. *American Journal of Psychiatry*, 165(5): 631–638.
Bion, W. (1961). *Experiences in groups*. London: Tavistock Publications.
Brown, D. (2006). Self-development through subjective interaction: A fresh look at ′ego training in action′. In J. Maratos (Ed.), *Resonance and Reciprocity: Selected Papers by Dennis Brown* (pp. 107–123). London: Routledge.
Brown, D. G. (1994). Self-development through subjective interaction: A fresh look at ′ego training in action′. In D. G. Brown & L. M. Zinkin (Eds.), *The Psyche and the Social World: Developments in Group Analytic Theory*. London: Routledge.
Esposito, G., Formentin, S., Marogna, C., et al. (2022). Pseudomentalization as a challenge for therapists of group psychotherapy with drug addicted patients. *Frontiers in Psychology*, 12(5432).
Folmo, E. J., Karterud, S. W., Bremer, K., et al. (2017). The design of the MBT-G adherence and quality scale. *Scandinavian Journal of Psychology*, 58(4): 341–349.
Fonagy, P., Campbell, C. & Bateman, A. (2017). Mentalizing, attachment, and epistemic trust in group therapy. *International Journal of Group Psychotherapy*, 67(2): 176–201.
Fonagy, P., Gergely, G., Jurist, E., et al. (2002). *Affect Regulation, Mentalization and the Development of the Self*. New York: Other Press.
Foulkes, S. H. (1948). *Introduction to Group Analytic Psychotherapy*. London: Karnac.
Foulkes, S. H. (1977). Notes on the concept of resonance. In L. R. Wolberg & M. L. Aronson (Eds.), *Group Therapy. An Overview* (pp. 52–58). New York: Stratton Intercontinental Medical Book Corporation.
Harrison, T. (2000). *Bion, Rickman, Foulkes and the Northfield Experiments. Advancing on a Different Front*. London, Philadelphia: Jessica Kingsley.
Hecke, D., Brand, T., Rietz, C., et al. (2016). Prozess-Outcome-Studie zum Gruppenklima in psychodynamischer (PDGT) und mentalisierungsbasierter Gruppenpsychotherapie (MBT-G) in einem tagesklinischen Setting – Was verändert wen? *Gruppenpsychother Gruppendynamik*, 52(2): 175–193.
Heigl-Evers, A. & Heigl, F. (1973). Gruppentherapie: Interaktionell – tiefenpsychologisch fundiert (analytisch orientiert) – psychoanalytisch. *Gruppenpsychother Gruppendynamik*, 7: 132–157.
Hummelen, B., Wilberg, T. & Karterud, S. (2007). Interviews of female patients with borderline personality disorder who dropped out of group psychotherapy. *International Journal of Group Psychotherapy*, 57(1): 67–91.
Inderhaug, T. & Karterud, S. (2015). A qualitative study of a mentalization-based group for borderline patients. *Group Analysis*, 48(2): 150–163.
Jones, M. (1963). The therapeutic community. In A. Deutsch & H. Fishman (Eds.), *The Encyclopedia of Mental Health* (pp. 1992–1996). London: Franklin Watts.
Karterud, S. (1998). The group, self, empathy. Intersubjectivity and hermeneutics: A group analytic perspective. In I. Harwood & M. Pines (Eds.), *Self Experiences in Groups. Intersubjective and Self Psychological Pathways to Human Understanding* (pp. 83–98). London: Jessica Kingsley Publishers.

Karterud, S. (2011). Constructing and mentalizing the matrix. *Group Analysis,* 44(4): 357–373.
Karterud, S. (2012). *Manual for mentaliseringsbasert gruppeterapi (MBT-G).* Oslo: Gyldendal Akademisk.
Karterud, S. (2015a). *Mentalization-Based Group Therapy (MBT-G).* Oxford: Oxford University Press.
Karterud, S. (2015b). On structure and leadership in mentalization-based group therapy and group analysis. *Group Analysis,* 48(2): 137–149.
Karterud, S. (2018). Case formulations in mentalization-based group therapy. *Research in Psychotherapy: Psychopathology, Process and Outcome,* 21: 132–136.
Karterud, S., Folmo, E. & Kongerslev, M. T. (2019). Personality and the group matrix. *Group Analysis,* 52(4): 503–519.
Karterud, S., Vaglum, S., Friis, S., et al. (1992). Day hospital therapeutic community treatment for patients with personality disorders. An empirical evaluation of the containment function. *Journal of Nervous and Mental Disease,* 180(4): 238–243.
Kohut, H. (1971). *The analysis of the self.* New York: International Universities Press.
Kvarstein, E. H., Pedersen, G., Urnes, O., et al. (2015). Changing from a traditional psychodynamic treatment programme to mentalization-based treatment for patients with borderline personality disorder--does it make a difference? *Psychology and Psychotherapy,* 88(1): 71–86.
Marziali, E. & Munroe-Blum, H. (1994). *Interpersonal Group Psychotherapy for Borderline Personality Disorder.* New York: Basic Books.
Morken, K. T. E., Binder, P.-E., Arefjord, N. M., et al. (2019). Mentalization-based treatment from the patients' perspective – what ingredients do they emphasize? *Frontiers in Psychology,* 10.
Nitsun, M. (2014 [1996]). *The Anti-Group – Destructive Forces in the Group and Their Creative Potential.* London: Routledge.
Pines, M. (1990). Group analytic psychotherapy and the borderline patient. In B. E. Roth, W. N. Stone, & H. D. Kibel (Eds.), *The Difficult Patient in Group: Group Psychotherapy with Borderline and Narcissistic Disorders* (pp. 31–44). Madison: International University Press.
Schlapobersky, J. (2016). *From the Couch to the Circle: Group-Analytic Psychotherapy in Practice.* London: Routledge.
Schultz-Venrath, U. (2022). Es begann in Amerika …- die USA als Entstehungsort von Gruppenanalyse und Gruppensychotherapie. In G. Dietrich & F. Fossel (Eds.), *Gruppenpsychoanalyse – Theorie, Geschichte und Praxisfelder der gruppenanalytischen Methode* (pp. 151–167). Wien: Facultas.
Schultz-Venrath, U. & Felsberger, H. (2016). *Mentalisieren in Gruppen.* Stuttgart: Klett-Cotta.
Staats, H. (2010). Combining individual and group therapy in an out-patient setting for patients with personality disorders – useful approach or invitation to acting out? In A. M. Schloesser & A. Gerlach (Eds.), *Crossing Borders – Integrating Differences: Psychoanalytic Psychotherapy in Transition* (pp. 39–54). London: Karnac.
Staats, H., Bolm, T. & Dally, A. (2014). Das Göttinger Modell der Gruppenpsychotherapie. In H. Staats, A. Dally, & T. Bolm (Eds.), *Gruppenpsychotherapie und Gruppenanalyse. Ein Lehr-und Lernbuch für Klinik und Praxis* (pp. 47–56). Göttingen: Vandenhoeck & Ruprecht.

Stanghellini, G. (2017). *Lost in Dialogue.* Oxford: Oxford University Press.
Whitaker, D. S. & Lieberman, M. (1964). *Psychotherapy through the Group Process.* Chicago: Atherton Press.
Wu, H., Liu, X., Hagan, C. C. & Mobbs, D. (2020). Mentalizing during social InterAction: A four component model. *Cortex*. 126: 242–252.

Chapter 11

Mentalizing and group analysis in development

Sigmund Karterud

Abstract

In the first chapter, I conducted a discussion about the very concept of mentalizing and the challenges of group analysis to live up to its theoretical and therapeutic potentials. The following articles, covering the years 2003–2024, illustrate the conceptual, historical and therapeutic processes which has coined MBT-G and group analysis, led them apart, while also inviting them for a closer collaboration. In this final chapter, I summarise the development of these ideas.

It starts with the self (Karterud & Stone, 2003) and with reference to the pioneer Heinz Kohut, the founder of psychoanalytic self psychology. The self is the experiential centre of the person and the source of his/her emotions, actions and relations. All psychotherapies should be grounded upon a valid theory of the self. Unfortunately, that is not always the case. Kohut's self was not the ultimate answer. However, it was a crucial starting point. Today we will reconceptualise some of his tenets. I fully endorse the concept of basic needs of the self, in order to develop and thrive, and thereby the concept of selfobjects. However, I would downplay the concept of *mirroring* and highlight the concept of *being minded.* Being mirrored refers more to the emotional part of the self, while being minded refers more to the phenomenon of being understood which carry implicit references to the linguistic fabric of the surrounds and whereby the individual becomes integrated into the language speaking human community. Being minded comes with a stronger emphasis on the significance of self-consciousness. A qualitative study of a mentalization-based group for borderline patients. The ultimate aim of self-development, so to speak, is attainment of self-consciousness and that is a linguistic affair. It demands language, which in turns demands institutionalized groups. These implications were not elaborated in early self psychology. However, what was very much implicated was the significance of empathy. And indeed, empathy is a crucial component of the kind of minding that consolidates the self. Stating that the ultimate aim of self-development is self-consciousness, might seem like an exaggeration. And in a certain sense it is. The ultimate aim can also be phrased like becoming a healthy person that is capable of taking care of him/herself, his/her family and friends, and

DOI: 10.4324/9781003625810-11

the community to which he/she belongs. However, to realize such a life project, the person will need self-consciousness. And self-consciousness is not a thing. It is not an either or. It is a creative process of thinking, feeling and relating with the presupposition that it is ME that thinks, feels and relates in a manner which is beneficial for myself and my friends.

In a recent volume on ICD-11, Åse-Line Baltzersen (2025) has written a moving story about her personal journey from utterly confusion, chaos, fragmentation and destructiveness to restauration of the self through a treatment process where long-term group therapy was a major component. Finding and developing the inner core of herself was not the result of any particular interpretation or circumscribed event in the group. It was the long-term participation in a caring but challenging group that provoked a wide range of emotions and relational experiences which were thought about (minded) by the self-reflective group. Her story also underlines that it is not only to *verbalize* "autistic" parts of oneself which a superficial reading of Foulkes might suggest. When so-called "autistic" parts become verbalized, they also come with a lot of emotions, confusion, relational turmoil and difficulties with owning previously disavowed experiences. Baltzersen writes about a fragmented and disorganized self which is not able to find a meaningful way of living in the world and the long and strenuous process of recovery through the group processes. It is about integrating contradictory parts of the self and developing new capabilities.

The story of Åse-Line Baltzersen describes the process of developing increased self-consciousness, meaning that the person has come to own her different self-states as HERS, and taken the responsibility of them in ways of living with others. Our article (Karterud & Stone, 2003) describes how the concepts from self psychology help the therapist in creating a group culture that can sustain such a restorative process. The article was written at a time before Searle had fully developed his theory of social ontology, i.e., the significance of constitutive speech act declarations that come with deontological power. However, the elaboration of the group self is fully compatible with Searle. In our terminology we define the essence of the group self as located in its "project" (constitutive speech act declaration) and that this project set the "tone" of the group, by which we mean the group discourse that develops and its supra-individual nature. Or to cite ourselves: "The nature of the project defines the kind of discourse that is most appropriate for the group". We then proceed to describe the selfobject function of this discourse as a means for creativity and development of the self that transcends individual reflections and two-person conversations when it is performed successfully. In addition, we highlight the significance of sheer otherness. By that time, these ideas were not yet integrated with the theory of mentalizing which was published in 2002 (Fonagy et al., 2002). That was a task for the coming years. There was something in development.

In Chapter three, in the paper on group dreams (Stone & Karterud, 2006), we incorporate aspects of mentalizing theory to understand the nature of dream mentation. It is not linear and logical deductive. In groups, the sensory qualities are palpable and strange plots based upon visual images play a greater role than verbal discourse. It testifies of more primitive modes of thinking, including psychic equivalence and pretend mode in another kind of consciousness than the ordinary self-conscious state of the individual. In a tribute to Freud, we emphasize for psychotherapy group members that dreams are the best proof of the significance of deeper strata of the mind. In modern terms we do not say that dreams attest to repressed and unconscious plots that should be made conscious. Rather we say that dreams attest to unmentalized or poorly mentalized personal experiences from the past that influence upon experiences in present day life, which includes the life in the group which gradually will be more and more emotionally significant for the participants. Thus, dream mentation may be seen as a source of making sense of the present in the light of the past. We also underline the creative aspect of dreams in that they may point at new possibilities for being in the world through the dream imaginaries. We refer here to Marian Tolpin's theory of the quest for self-development ("the forward edge") when self-protective barriers start to decline. We argue that a strong emphasis on group dreams should be a hallmark of a mature therapeutic group self (discourse).

In Chapter four, the 2012 Foulkes lecture "Constructing and mentalizing the matrix", steps are taken towards an integration of mentalizing theory and group analysis. Critics might say at the expense of group analysis. And I partly agree. However, it was not done for ideological reasons. The paper describes in detail the experimentations and research that guided our new ways of conducting groups for (mostly) borderline patients. The foundation for this research was the Norwegian Network for Day Hospital Treatment (later renamed The Norwegian Network for Personality Disorder) which we founded in 1992. It has counted around 20 group therapy units from all over Norway, using the same test procedures for assessment, treatment course, outcome and follow up (Pedersen et al., 2022). Due to the sheer number of groups, patients and outcome data we were able to empirically assess the results of different group therapy approaches and techniques. Regrettable, such an empirical approach to dynamic group psychotherapy had previously been lacking in group analytic communities. Based upon these empirical data, extensive video studies and discussions among competent peers, we finally came to agreement about therapeutic principles for psychotherapy with groups where most members suffered a personality disorder (Karterud, 2015). These innovations were created in a perpetual dialogue with group analysis. The overriding topic was the concept of group matrix, as the title "Constructing and mentalizing the matrix" suggests. In classical group analysis the matrix evolves seemingly spontaneously due to the interactions between the group members and the interpretive and analytic interventions of the group analyst. In MBT group therapy, the therapist(s) take a more active role in structuring the matrix through psychoeducation and explicit suggestions about structure and means to achieve the goals of the groups which is self- and personality development.

The article in Chapter 5, "A qualitative study of a mentalization-based group for borderline patients" (Inderhaug & Karterud, 2015), illustrates the empirical approach towards a broader implementation of MBT-G in the health care system. We made a detailed study of three consecutive video-recorded group therapy sessions in a mental health centre in the middle region of Norway. We were surprised to find the same chaotic group processes that MBT was designed to prevent. It provided a good opportunity to investigate what went wrong. Our study of the video and the transcripts (59.000 words) revealed that the therapists failed to undertake an authoritative role and that they overplayed the principle of not-knowing stance. It gave us an opportunity to clarify these issues.

Chapter 6, "On structure and leadership in mentalization-based group therapy and group analysis" (Karterud, 2015), conducts a wider discussion on the problems as revealed in Chapter 5. It provides strong arguments for transcending the previous object-relational paradigm of group analysis. Mentalizing is something more than object relations. It concerns the fabric of the self and the person's capacity for feeling, thinking and relating. As I write in the introduction to the chapter where I highlight that prerequisites for sound social cognition,

> are likely to become violated when the communicational re-education take place in a group composed of personality disordered individuals who receive minimal instructions on how to proceed. Such experiments likely end up in disconnected speech and utterances, aborted stories conveying fragments of experience, emotional outbursts and activation of psychic equivalence, malign projective identifications, sequences of pseudomentalization, experiences of not being heard and respected, as well hopelessness and disillusionment as demonstrated in several of the citations in the article of Inderhaug & Karterud (2015). Such situations call for therapists, not as conductors, but as competent leaders who model a kind of parental-like authority. This parental-like authority is less concerned with what is right or wrong, as how to reach truth about oneself and others. Philosophically, such an attitude is grounded in communicational ethics (e.g., Grice, 1989; Habermas, 1984), which concerns the implicit ethos of communication between humans, e.g., a wish for communication and conveying honest messages, a concern for truth, a respect for the dialog partner, active listening and an effort to understand the partner's mental state and point of view, etc. This kind of communication does not come by nature. It is hard won achievements of cultural (group) evolution. The concept of mentalizing stance belongs to this tradition of ideas.

And furthermore: Basically, the idea is that by the individual group members striving to become a member of the mentalizing group self, i.e. the work group aspect of the group, one has to develop one's social cognition (Karterud & Stone, 2003). Or phrased in another way: The development of social cognition (narration, attention, focusing, inhibitory control, affect consciousness, metacognition, mentalizing, integration, etc.) is likely to be a result of one's efforts to become a member of the group self. This logic is supported by modern theories of evolution of thinking, self-consciousness and culture (Bogdan, 2013; Tomasello, 2019).

Chapter 7, "A comparative study mentalization-based versus psychodynamic group therapy" (Kalleklev & Karterud, 2018) demonstrates the necessity of an empirical research approach to group dynamics. At this stage we were well versed in the use of the MBT adherence and competence scale (MBT-ACS) since it had been implemented as a routine instrument for quality control at the MBT Laboratory of Oslo University Hospital. In this study we combined it with the Reflective Functioning (RF) scale developed by Fonagy and coworkers. A superficial judgement of the video recordings of the groups under study, one MBT group and one psychodynamic group, would presumably say that these groups were pretty much alike. However, the careful ratings of the therapist's interventions and the course of RF of the protagonist members of these groups revealed substantial differences. The in-session outcome was that the protagonists in the MBT group increased their ability for reflective functioning (mentalizing) while the protagonists in the psychodynamic group did not. Our data suggested that the differences were due to interventions (speech acts) of the therapists in the MBT group which more often were of a "demand question" (challenging) type while the interventions in the psychodynamic group were mostly supportive. The implications for quality control and training of group therapists are substantial. They point to the need for video recordings and rating scales for detecting crucial nuances in the group discourse.

Chapter 8, "A high-quality mentalization-based group therapy session" (Karterud, 2018), provides more substance to the preceding remarks on empirical process research. It builds on the previous paper and present a graphic therapist intervention profile as well as a thorough group transcript where the therapist's interventions are rated according to the MBT-G-ACS. The transcript reveals the substantial increase in reflective functioning of the protagonist, the constructive contributions from the other group members and the significance of the demand questions of the therapists.

The article in chapter 9, "Personality and the group matrix" (Karterud, Folmo & Kongerslev, 2019) refers to the tripartite conception of the matrix theory, as discussed by Nitzgen and Hopper (2017). We maintain that the personal matrix has been grossly neglected and shortly describe the temperament-attachment-mentalizing (TAM) theory of personality (Karterud & Kongerslev, 2019) which might enrich group analysis as well as mentalizing theory. We also uphold the relevance of entropy theory since groups are social systems that require energy for their boundary maintenance. Devoid of such energy, groups will dissolve. This view is compatible with the social ontology theory of Searle where the energy is conceived as the deontological power that follows the constitutive declarations of groups. The thesis is substantiated by a study of a video-recorded group where the group matrix was energized by the therapists for the first 60 minutes, displaying a high-quality discourse in a group with mainly personality disorders, while thereafter collapsing into ordinary social talk.

Chapter 10 (Karterud et al., 2024) has a more historic flavour. It describes the challenges for group analysis as a mode of group psychotherapy around the millennium and the rise of MBT as a competing therapy when it comes to personality disorders. Unfortunately, the competing elements have been pervasive from both sides. Especially in the UK while in other countries, like Norway and Germany, there have been friendly cooperation and exchange of views. The paper strongly recommends more cooperation, to the benefit of both parties.

Altogether, this volume describes a field in perpetual development. Hopefully I have succeeded in describing how this development has been influenced by new ideas in philosophy, the science of evolution, neurobiology and affective neuroscience, developmental psychology, the theory of mentalizing, new conceptualizations of personality and its disorders, new technologies for measuring individual and group processes alongside with therapeutic innovations and a general move away from metapsychology and towards empirical research. The main influence though has come from the theory of mentalizing. These trends have also been influenced by changes in the Zeitgeist and the way mental health services are organised in Western countries with a strong emphasis on so-called evidence-based psychotherapies. These developments will continue and hopefully this volume represents a fruitful contribution for further theoretical integration and for the quality of group psychotherapy as a clinical practice.

References

Baltzersen, Å. L. (2025). A lived experience and recovery perspective. In B. Bach (Ed.), *ICD-11 Personality Disorders. Assessment and Treatment*. Oxford: Oxford University Press.

Bogdan, R. J. (2013). *Mindvaults: The Sociocultural Grounds for Pretending and Imagining*. Cambridge: MIT Press.

Fonagy, P., Gergely, G., Jurist, E. L. & Target, M. (2002). *Affect Regulation, Mentalization, and the Development of the Self*. New York: Other Press.

Grice, P. (1989). *Studies in the Way of Words*. London: Harvard University Press.

Habermas, J. (1984). *The Theory of Communicative Action*. Boston: Beacon Press.

Inderhaug, T. & Karterud, S. (2015) A qualitative study of a mentalization-based group for borderline patients, *Group Analysis*, 48(2): 150–163.

Kalleklev, J. & Karterud, S. (2018). A comparative study of a mentalization-based versus a psychodynamic group therapy session. *Group Analysis*, 51(1): 44–60.

Karterud, S. (2015) On structure and leadership in MBT-G and group analysis. *Group Analysis*, 48(2): 137–149.

Karterud, S. (2018). A high-quality mentalization-based group therapy session. *Group Analysis*, 51(1): 18–43.

Karterud, S. (2015). *Mentalization-Based Group Therapy (MBT-G). A Theoretical, Clinical and Research Manual.* London: Oxford University Press.

Karterud, S. & Kongerslev, M. T. (2019). A Temperament, Attachment and Mentalization-based (TAM) theory of personality and its disorders. *Frontiers in Psychology*, 10: 518.

Karterud, S. & Stone, W. N. (2003). The group self: A neglected aspect of group psychotherapy. *Group Analysis,* 36(1): 7–22.

Karterud, S., Folmo, E. & Kongerslev, M. T. (2019). Personality and the group matrix. *Group Analysis*, 52(4), 503–519.

Karterud, S., Gunnarsen, G., Kongerslev, M. T., Staun, L. & Schultz-Venrath, U. (2024). On the relationship between group analysis and mentalization-based group therapy. *Group Analysis*, 58(1), 115–129.

Nitzgen, D. & Hopper, E. (2017). The concepts of the social unconscious and of the matrix in the work of S. H. Foulkes. In Hopper, E. & Weiberg, H. (Eds.), *The Social Unconsciousnes in Persons, Groups, and Societies: The Foundation Matrix Extended and Re-Configured.* London: Karnac Books.

Pedersen, G., Wilberg, T., Hummelen, B. & Kvarstein, E. (2023). The Norwegian network for personality disorders – development, contributions and challenges through 30 years. *Nordic Journal of Psychiatry*, 77(5): 512–520.

Stone, W. N, & Karterud, S. (2006). Dreams as portraits of self and group interaction. *International Journal of Group Psychotherapy*, 56(1): 47–62.

Tomasello, M. (2019). *Becoming Human: A Theory of Ontogeny.* Cambridge: Belknap Press.

Index